Ultimate

Core Ball

Workout

Strengthening and Sculpting Exercises with over 200 Step-by-Step Photos

JEANINE DETZ

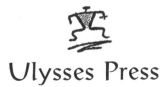

Ulysses Press

Published in the United States by
Ulysses Press
P.O. Box 3440
Berkeley, CA 94703
www.ulyssespress.com

ISBN 1-56975-468-3
Library of Congress Control Number 2005922424

Printed in Canada by Transcontinental Printing

10 9 8 7 6 5 4 3 2 1

Editorial/Production	Lily Chou, Claire Chun, Steven Zah Schwartz
	Tamara Kowalski
Design	Sarah Levin
Index	Sayre Van Young
Photography	Robert Holmes
Models	Jeanine Detz, Melanie Clifford, Kelly Keen, Diego Schmunis

Distributed in the United States by Publishers Group West
and in Canada by Raincoast Books

Please Note

This book has been written and published strictly for informational purposes, and in no way
should be used as a substitute for consultation with health care professionals. You should not
consider educational material herein to be the practice of medicine or to replace consultation
with a physician or other medical practitioner. The author and publisher are providing you
with information in this work so that you can have the knowledge and can choose, at your
own risk, to act on that knowledge. The author and publisher also urge all readers to be
aware of their health status and to consult health care professionals before beginning any
health program.

ACKNOWLEDGEMENTS

I'd like to thank everyone at Ulysses Press, especially Ashley, for bringing this project to me,
and Lily and Claire, for their hard work and support. Special thanks to the models for their
time and skill, and Robert Holmes for his talent and humor. Thanks to Steve Stiefel for his
support, insight and, most of all, faith in my ability. And finally, thanks to my family: Steve,
Lee, Chris, Neil, Jenna and Jamie, for their love and support.

contents

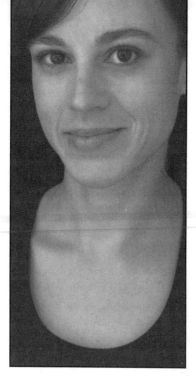

introduction

Whether you exercise regularly and want to increase your core strength, are on a weight-loss program, are new to exercise, are a senior who is looking for a modified program or are a new mom who is finding it difficult to regain her pre-pregnancy body, the *Ultimate Core Ball Workout* is for you. This book will give you all the information you need to strengthen the muscles of your abdominals and back. A strong core can decrease back pain, improve posture and (perhaps most desirable) make you look better.

You've already taken the first step toward attaining the benefits of a strengthened core: You purchased this book. With a small investment in time spent reading these pages, you'll be rewarded with the results you desire. Even if you've exercised for years, I urge you to follow this book and the steps within it carefully. After all, if you knew everything there was to know about core training, you wouldn't have picked up this book! As a fitness writer and editor, I sometimes think there's nothing new to learn about exercise, but am consistently surprised to take away new information from every project I work on. This one was no different. It's my sincere hope that it provides you with an enjoyable and effective guide to sculpting your core.

How This Book Is Organized

This book is designed to make the process of sculpting your core easy, efficient and enjoyable. In this first section, I introduce you to core training on the ball and explain all the tools you'll need to be successful in your pursuit. You'll learn a bit about the anatomy of your core—which muscles make up that part of your body and how they're involved in your every-day movements—and why the ball is such an effective tool for training these body parts. Next I explain the terms and techniques used throughout the book to ensure that you know what I'm talking about when I tell you to "sit upright on the ball" or "stabilize your back," for example. You'll also find some suggestions on how to purchase the right ball for your body, and other inexpensive equipment that will make your workouts even more effective. The section ends with an important chapter on how to combine the *Ultimate Core Ball Workout* with the other components of health and fitness to truly get the best results.

In Part 2, you'll find workouts composed of the exercises in the section that follows. I've purposely put the cart before the horse because I didn't want you to be tempted to jump into performing exercises without having an organized plan. That's because exercise order can be as important as the actual exercises. The workouts are divided into three levels of difficulty and you'll find detailed instructions to help you decide which level you're currently at and when to advance to the next one.

Part 3 is the nuts and bolts of this book: the exercises. There's more than 45 of them, and nothing is left to chance or guesswork. The instructions and photographs will take you through every step, ensuring that you're getting the most out

of each movement by doing it correctly. Also in the third part of the book are eight stretches that will become the basis of your cool-downs. Again, there will be no guesswork. From step-by-step instructions to suggestions for modifications, everything you need to relax and stretch the muscles you've worked is included.

Before You Get Started

Before beginning the *Ultimate Core Ball Workout* or any exercise program, consult with a doctor or physician. Ask him or her to evaluate your current health, and to recommend precautions you should take in your fitness program. If you have an existing injury, have it evaluated and follow the beginner variations for exercises that might aggravate it.

If you experience any pain while doing the exercises in this book, you are not working correctly. Immediately stop, reread the directions and try the move again with less intensity. If an exercise is painful, don't do it.

CAUTION: The exercises in this book are NOT intended, and may be dangerous, for pregnant women since they focus on the abdominals and require you to compress the abdominal wall. Post-natal women should receive clearance from their doctor before beginning this or any exercise program. (Most physicians recommend you avoid strenuous exercise for at least 6 to 8 weeks after giving birth, longer if you had a Caesarean section.)

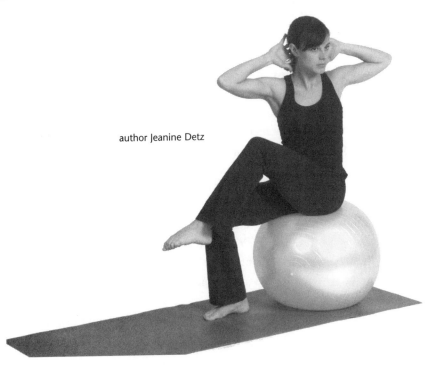

author Jeanine Detz

get to the core

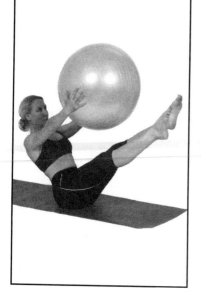

"Core" has become a fitness buzz word. From Pilates and ballet-inspired workouts to sports conditioning, everyone is telling you to work your core. Before you learn why that's important, first get your anatomy straight and figure out what exactly that ubiquitous "core" is.

Many people believe that only the muscles of their abdomen make up their core, but that's a misnomer. When we refer to the "core," we're talking about the muscles of your abdominals and lower back. Imagine wrapping a girdle around your lower torso—everything it covers, or holds in, from front to back is your core. These muscles are engaged and support your body in nearly every endeavor, from sitting at a desk to running a marathon. This section explores the muscles of each group and their function in your body. Before you read on, or skip this chapter and move on to the exercises, I'd like to point out that you don't need to memorize where muscles originate or

their exact location in your body. Exercise doesn't require a degree. However, you will get more out of your workouts with some basic knowledge about what you're working. That's the purpose of this section, and it's an important one.

Abdominals

The abdominals (or "abs") are composed of four muscle groups: rectus abdominis, external obliques, internal obliques and transverse abdominis.

The **rectus abdominis** is the group that most people think of when they refer to abdominals. It's the muscle that runs from your pubic bone to your sternum (breastbone) and it gives you the coveted "six-pack" definition. When you bend forward,

the rectus abdominis does most of the flexing. This muscle group also tilts the pelvis. The rectus abdominis is activated in nearly every exercise in this book, as it's impossible to isolate when you're working other body parts.

The **external obliques** are the muscles that run diagonally downward from your lower ribs to the top of your pelvic bone. They are attached to the rectus abdominis by connective tissue. Since these muscles assist in twisting your torso, they are worked hardest during side-to-side movements.

You also have **internal obliques**, which run diagonally upward from your pelvic bone to your lower ribs and are located beneath your external obliques. These muscles assist the external obliques in twisting movements.

The **transverse abdominis** runs from front to back, attaches to the lower ribs and the spine, then runs horizontally to attach to the connective tissue of the rectus abdominis. It's located underneath the obliques. It's the deepest of the abdominal muscles and it contracts when the other muscles of the abdominals are working, pulling the abdominals inward.

Lower Back

The **latissimus dorsi** is a large triangular-shaped muscle that attaches at the top of your hipbone, extends over the lower and middle back, and attaches at the rear of your upper arm. This muscle moves your arms behind you and helps your shoulders rotate.

The **erector spinae** is a muscle group made up of three muscle pairs called spine extensors. They run the entire length of your spine on either side and attach at your ribs and spine. The erector spinae work to keep your spine upright in nearly every movement.

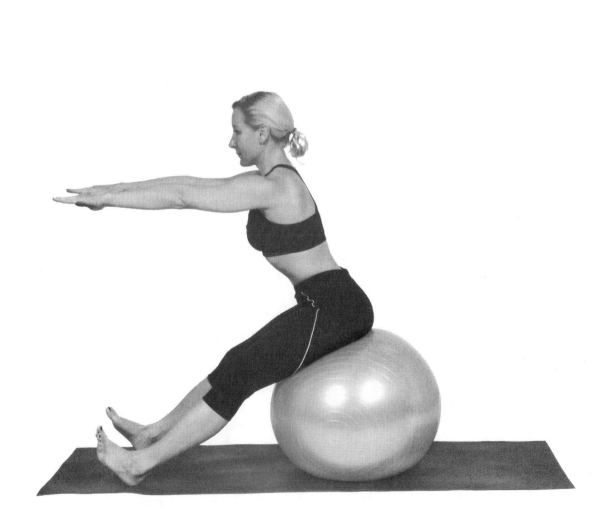

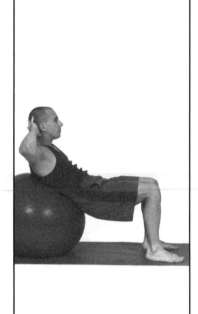

working the core: why the ball?

During the past several years, people have begun to better understand the link between weak core muscles, back pain and poor posture. Because of this, there's been a strong increase in core training. However, most people never get the results they want. The reason? They are misinformed and are training their cores ineffectively.

Every time I go to the gym or take a fitness class, I'm amazed (and saddened) by the number of people who are still doing endless crunches in hopes that they'll get the midsection of their dreams.

If you're short on time (and really, who isn't?) or are simply looking to train your core in a more efficient manner (and obviously you are), then the stability ball is your perfect core training companion. Sit on one of these rubber wonders, place your hands on your abs, and you'll immediately discover the benefits. Since the ball is an unstable surface, it forces your abs to engage to keep you in a seated, upright position. What's more, those deepest muscles of your abs—the transverse abdominis—are recruited.

If you doubt that merely sitting on one of these balls works your abs, try this experiment: Sit on the ball for a half-hour. Don't do any exercises, just sit—you can watch TV, read or work on your computer—but the key is to just be seated in an upright position. The next day, your abs will be sore, indicating they were worked. Now if you can work your core by merely sitting on a ball, imagine what can happen when you perform exercises on one. You actually don't have to imagine how much more effective the exercises will be—someone has gone ahead and researched it.

In a study performed in the Health Sciences department at Springfield College in Springfield, Massachusetts, researchers compared the effects of exercises performed on the ball to those compared on the floor. One group of women performed

CORE FUNCTIONS

Your core muscles serve as both movers and stabilizers, and you can work those muscles with stabilization exercises and movement exercises. Both entail what their names suggest. *Stabilization* exercises require you to hold your body in a position, which forces your muscles to contract to keep the body still or balanced. *Movement* exercises engage your muscles by making them move your body. This book includes both types of exercises (and many that are a combination of the two) because it's important to work your muscles the way they function.

two exercises on a ball; the other performed them on the floor. After five weeks, the group that had worked on the ball had greater gains in torso balance, as well as back and abdominal stability, than the floor exercise group. [*The Journal of Strength and Conditioning Research* (Vol. 17, No. 3, Aug. 2003)]

Besides the important function of instantly engaging your core muscles and keeping them engaged, the ball has several other benefits in your training. First, when performing many of the exercises in this book, the spherical shape of the ball forces you to work the abs through a full range of motion. For example, when you do a crunch on the floor or other flat surface, the distance you move is limited. However, when you do the same exercise on the ball, your body can extend farther forward and back. This means your abs are worked through a fuller range of motion.

Another benefit of the ball for core training is that it forces you to work a bit slower than you would on the floor. Think about it: If you raise and lower your body quickly on the ball, you'll fall over. Moving through exercises more slowly means that the muscles are contracted for a longer period of time, which, of course, translates into a tougher workout.

Although this book focuses on your core, the truth is, you'll be working other parts of your body as well. That's because working on the ball doesn't fully isolate your core. When you're performing a seated exercise, your thighs will be engaged to hold the ball in place. When you're doing inverted movements, such as the Knee Tuck from Plank, your shoulders and arms will be working. A mobile surface like the ball forces the muscles of your back, hips, legs and arms to focus on the movement. So be prepared to see improvements in every part of your body, not just your core.

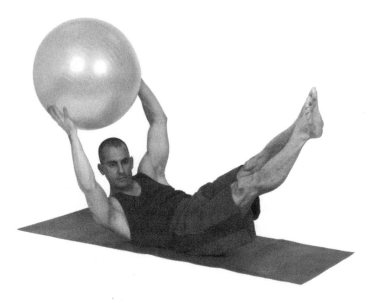

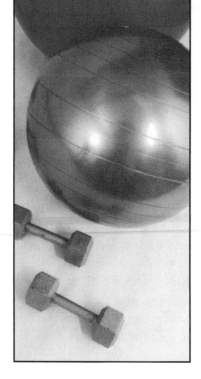

equip yourself

If you have a stability ball, a floor to place it on and a little bit of space to maneuver around in, you're ready to do the exercises in this book. There are some additional items, however, that will make your workout more comfortable, challenging and safe.

Don't worry, they won't add much to your expenses, and that brings me to one more point. One of the many excuses I hear from people who don't exercise—especially those who live in big cities like my own— is that it costs too much to join a gym. The truth is, for about what you'd spend on a one-month gym membership, you can purchase everything you need to get in shape. In this section, I outline everything you need to effectively work your core, dedication not included.

Ball

Stability balls (also called Swiss, exercise and balance balls) can be found in nearly every sports equipment store, as well as at discount retailers and on websites. A stability ball typically costs between $15 and $50. While you may be tempted to just buy the first, or cheapest, one you find, there are some important points to keep in mind. First, durability. Most stability balls are made of comparable-weight heavy plastic that will resist wear and tear for at least a year. For this reason, you don't necessarily have to buy a more expensive ball to get an effective one.

Next, size. Stability balls typically come in three sizes, one of which will be appropriate for you. Size recommendations vary by source. I've found that the following general guidelines, dispensed by the American Council on Exercise, are most

HEIGHT/BALL DIAMETER	
less than 5'	45 cm
5' to 5'7"	55 cm
5'7" TO 6'2"	65 cm
over 6'2"	75 cm

accurate. Find your height to determine which size ball you should purchase. If you fall at the cutoff for a size, you may have to try one or two to find a comfortable fit. Remember, you can always deflate the ball and return it if it isn't a good fit.

Which brings me to my next point: fit. Inflate the ball (most manufacturers now include a hand or foot pump, but you can also use an air compressor or bicycle pump) and sit on top of it, with your bottom firmly planted in its center. In this position, your legs should be bent at about a 90-degree angle and your thighs should be parallel to the floor. If your knees are higher than your hips and come up toward your chest, the ball is too small. If your hips are higher than your knees and feel like they're rolled forward, the ball is too large. This is also a good time to check the air pressure.

Your weight should press the ball down slightly but noticeably. If it doesn't, deflate it a bit. If it's mushy beneath you, add more air. You may also want to make sure that the ball is inflated fully by measuring it. Here's how: Let's say you purchased a ball that's 65cm in diameter. With a tape measure, calculate 65cm from the floor and mark that on a wall. Push the ball against the wall and place a ruler at its highest point. It should hit the mark. This all may sound a tedious, but taking the right precautions will ensure your workouts are comfortable, injury-free and effective. Once you've found the right ball, take care of it. Store it in a clean area out of direct sunlight or heat (both can damage the ball's plastic surface). Don't let pets or children play with it. If the ball collects dirt, clean it with a cloth dampened with warm, soapy water. (Don't hose it down, as water might enter and compromise its shape or durability.)

Mat

While you can do many of these exercises with the ball on a carpeted or bare floor, I think you'll find the grip of a mat helpful. A yoga mat, or other thin rubber exercise mat, creates a more stable surface for the ball and also provides a bit of cushioning for those times when you lose your balance. (Trust me, they'll happen!) You'll also find a mat useful for exercises done with your back on the floor. Opt for a thinner mat over a thicker one, as they tend to be less obtrusive and store more easily.

Room to Work

Sure, the ball doesn't take up much space, but you'll need a good clear perimeter around you to work out safely. I learned the importance of this point a few years ago while attempting to do yoga in my tiny apartment. I cleared out enough space for my mat, but as I stretched my arms down into a swan dive, my right arm didn't

quite clear the TV. I only bruised my hand, but it taught me an important lesson in safety. To be sure you have enough room to safely do the exercises in this book, clear out at least a mat's length of space in all directions. That way, if the ball slips out from under you, or you fall sideways, you won't run into any obstacles.

It's also helpful to have a clear wall space nearby. Leaning the ball against a wall for some of these exercises can make balance easier, especially if you're just starting out. A wall is required for some of the variations. Don't have clear wall space in your home? I can certainly relate. Just close a door between two rooms and use the back of the door as your "wall."

Weights

As you advance, you may need added resistance to make your core workouts more effective. Some of the exercise variations in this book call for the use of a dumbbell. However, these are

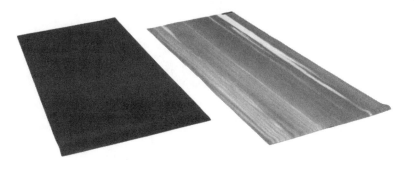

Sticky mats help prevent the ball from slipping.

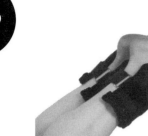

Ankle weights

only *options*. You really don't need weights to effectively work your core. If you choose to add weights, however, it's important to know that the core muscles don't require much to become fatigued. Therefore, purchase a

set of 3- or 5-pound dumbbells or a similar weighted medicine ball and you'll be set.

Clothing

You wouldn't wear tennis shoes and a tracksuit to a black-tie affair. Okay, some of you might, but my point is this: There are appropriate clothes for every event and activity, and exercise is no exception. You should wear comfortable clothing that allows unrestricted movement. You can wear pants or shorts, but you might find the latter a better choice if you're attempting exercises that require you to

have your legs on the ball. (Pants might cause slipping.) If you choose pants, make sure they're closer fitting. Your top should be comfortable, but not too loose. (It helps to see and feel your abs during many of the exercises.) You don't have to worry about shoes: The workouts in this book can be done with bare feet. In fact, unless you're in a gym where safety and hygiene are issues, I recommend bare feet. You'll find it easier to move through the positions and balance yourself in inverted positions without shoes.

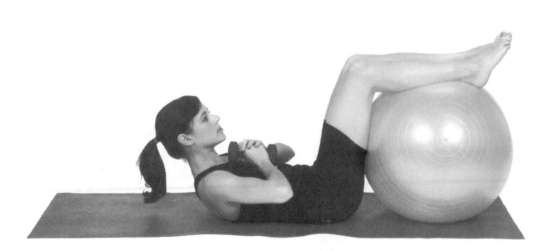

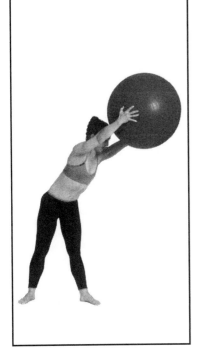

form follows function

You've heard the cliche "It's all in the technique" in reference to everything from cooking to sex. Nowhere is this maxim truer than in fitness. Learning the *right* way to work out will not only make your program more effective, it will also prevent injury. If you've been exercising for a while, you should already be familiar with some of the terms and techniques in this chapter. If you're just starting out, they may be entirely new to you. Whatever your experience level is, I guarantee you'll learn something new in the next few pages.

Sets and Reps

A repetition or "rep" is one complete exercise performed through its entire range of motion. For example, if you perform one ball crunch—raise yourself then lower yourself— you've completed one rep. A set is a number of reps performed consecutively. For example, if a workout tells you to do three sets of 10 knee raises, you'll do 30 raises total. You'll find these terms in the programs and exercises sections.

Frequency, Rest and Recovery

Muscles gain strength from use. (This is simple to understand when you consider what your abs look like after years without exercise!) The workouts in this book will be most effective when you do them two to three times per week. Many people don't realize that rest and recovery are equally important as frequency in your training. When you train your muscles, you're actually tearing their

fibers. Muscle growth occurs when those fibers rebuild. Rest is required for this rebuilding to occur. You should never train the same muscle group two days in a row. Many people disregard this recommendation when it comes to their abs, thinking that if they exercise the muscle group every day they'll see faster results. This isn't true. The muscles of your core, like every other group in your body, need at least 24 hours between training sessions

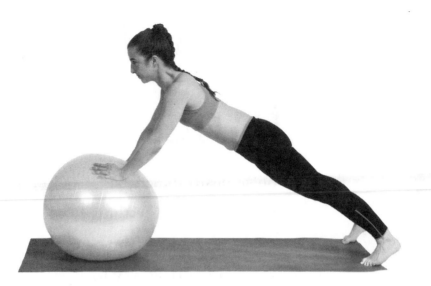

to recover and rebuild. Therefore, if you do a core workout on Monday, your next one shouldn't be done until Wednesday at the earliest.

Mixing It Up

At some point, you're going to hit a training plateau. It's a time when your progress seems to halt even though you've continued to train. The number one reason people hit such a stopping point is a lack of variation in their routine. When you first start doing a new exercise program, your body must adapt to it. During this adaptation, you'll make great gains in strength, performance and probably appearance. However, once your muscles get used to what you're doing, they'll no longer need to grow to adapt. This is when you reach a plateau, and where the importance of variety comes into play.

In order to continue spurring new growth, consistently change your exercise program. Every few weeks, you should change up any or all of the following variables: exercise order, type, intensity and frequency. The programs in this book have variation built right into them. When given an option for an exercise, simply choose a different one every week or so. Or sometimes do a specialized workout. Also remember to incorporate change into the other parts of your fitness program (cardiovascular and weight training) to achieve optimum results.

Soreness

Chances are you're going to experience muscle soreness at some time after doing the workouts in this book. If you've never exercised before, or it's been a while since you've worked out, you may be sore for the first few weeks. Be encouraged, not discouraged: Manageable soreness—the kind that doesn't impede your daily activities—is a sign that your workout challenged your muscles. Even if you've been exercising for years, you'll probably experience muscle soreness from these workouts because you're using your body in a new way.

If your abdominals are sore the day after your workout, and the soreness lasts up to a week, that's normal. If you have this type of soreness and it's time for your next workout, don't skip it! Instead, decrease the intensity. You can accomplish this by doing fewer reps or sets, eliminating the weight if you were using added resistance, or doing a less-intense version of an exercise. This strategy is called active recovery and it can decrease your soreness by forcing more blood to the affected area, encouraging repair and recovery.

Breathing

Of course you know how to breathe, but breathing during exercise is unique. When done correctly, it can help your muscles work more effectively, fuel you through a difficult workout and keep your muscles properly contracted. For all of the exercises in this book, you'll find directions on when to inhale and exhale during a movement. Generally it's best to inhale on the negative portion of an exercise (when you're relaxing the muscle) and exhale on the positive part of a movement (when you're contracting the working muscle the most). For example, when doing a crunch, you'll exhale as you lift your shoulder blades off the floor and inhale as you lower them back to the starting position. You should inhale through your nose and exhale through your mouth. I find that when I'm moving through a difficult point in an

exercise, fully exhaling out of my mouth really helps push me through it.

If you're just starting out, you may find it challenging to get the hang of exercising while concentrating on the inhale and exhale. That's okay; it's fine to breathe in your normal pattern until you get this one down. The most important thing to remember: Don't hold your breath.

Be Neutral

Throughout this book, I'll tell you to contract your abs to put your spine in a "neutral position." It's a term that's become second nature to me, but only after some practice. A neutral position for your core is one in which your lower back is naturally curved, not flattened or arched. This puts your pelvis in a safe, stress-free position and also activates your abs, particularly the transverse abdominis. Since every body is different, neutral spine position is something that varies from person to person.

You'll want to check your spinal form before every exercise to make sure your spine is in neutral. The exception is some of the floor exercises. For example, when you're lying on your back with your feet supported on the ball ("Crunch with Feet on Ball"), I'll tell you to press your lower back against the floor. That's because in positions such as that one, it's safer and less stressful for your back to be pressed down.

You need to keep your neck in a neutral position as well, especially when you're raising your torso from a reclined position. To maintain a neutral neck position, imagine holding an apple against your chest with your chin. This will help you sustain your head and neck alignment and prevent you from pulling on your neck.

Positioning Yourself

Throughout the exercise section, you will find some common starting positions for your body. Take a moment to familiarize yourself with the

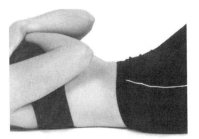

Incorrect Neutral Spine: Too Flat

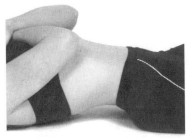

Incorrect Neutral Spine: Too Arched

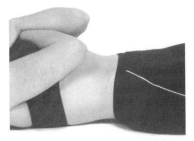

Correct Neutral Spine

following five, as they appear most often.

Sit Upright

When you're told to sit upright, it will be either on the floor or on top of the ball. Disregard your leg position for now and focus on the area of your body above your hips. When you're upright, the back of your head, shoulder blades and butt should be aligned. You may need to tighten your abs and push your hips slightly forward to properly set up in this position.

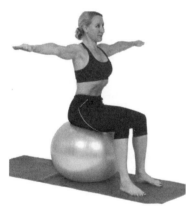

correct way to sit upright

Draw Your Shoulder Blades Down and Back

Stand sideways to a mirror, shrug your shoulders toward your ears and then slowly roll them back. You should see your shoulder blades push out like chicken wings. Next, from the pushed-back position, pull your shoulder blades down. This is "shoulder blades down and back" and it's the ideal starting point for many exercises since it stabilizes your upper body. It's also a critical component of sitting in an upright position.

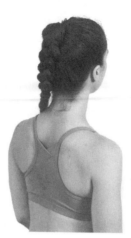

shoulders drawn and back

Drape Your Body Over the Ball

All of the exercises where you're face down on the ball begin with this instruction. It's simple to get into this position. Simply kneel behind the ball and hug it. Then roll your body slightly forward. You'll begin Plank from this relaxed position.

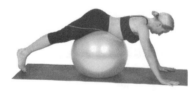

draping your body over the ball

Flex Your Feet

When your feet are flexed, their soles form 90- to 60-degree angles to your shins. To flex your feet, think about pulling the tops of them toward your legs.

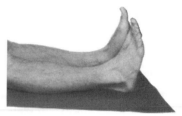

flexed feet

Point Your Feet

Pointing is the opposite of flexing. Think about pushing your toes (not bending them) toward your heels. You should feel the stretch and extension originating at the front of your ankles.

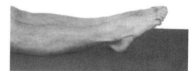

pointed feet

the big picture

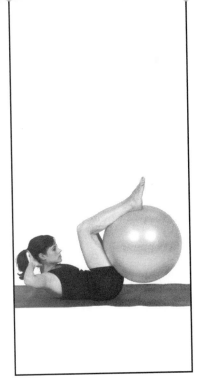

If you only do the workouts in this book as instructed, you'll see and feel improvements in the muscles of your abs and back, but you won't be fit. The reason? Your core is just one part of your body and strengthening exercises are just one part of fitness. Don't get me wrong: I strongly believe that core strength is extremely important. However, it's misleading and, quite frankly, wrong to imply that you'll get the midsection of your dreams without taking the other components of fitness into account. After all, if you have too much fat covering your abs, it doesn't matter how strong they are, they'll still look flabby.

To see marked improvements in your appearance and health, you need to include aerobic or cardiovascular exercise as well as strength training and stretching in your program. This chapter explains the importance of those components on your core as well as your total body fitness.

Nutrition

I don't have enough room here to go into the many intricacies of diet and nutrition. However, in some respects, all you need to know about dieting can be summed up in two sentences: If you take in more calories than you expend, you'll gain weight. If you burn more calories than you take in, you'll lose weight.

If you don't believe that, take a look at some of the more popular diets. I'll use low-carb as an example. Low-carb dieting involves cutting down on the amount of carbohydrate or starchy foods you eat and increasing the amount of protein you eat. When done in moderation, this is an effective weight-loss strategy. However, it's flawed in the assumption it causes many people to make: Carbohydrates are bad and make you gain weight. Like every other nutrient, there are "good" and "bad" carbohydrates. Low-carb diets usually involve cutting out refined or processed carbs that typically contain little fiber and nutritive value, and have lots of sugar and, thus, calories. Carbohydrates like fruits and vegetables, on the other hand, are an important part of a low-carb diet.

Although most people focus on nutrition only for weight loss, what you put into your body affects everything, from your mood and energy to your skin and hair. Eating well will maximize your workouts as well as your life. So starting today, stop viewing food as the enemy and start viewing it as your body does: fuel. If you have weight to lose, meet with a nutritionist to design a healthy meal plan. If you already eat well, congratulations. You're one step closer to total fitness and your ultimate core.

Cardio

Cardiovascular exercise is really any exercise that gets your heart pumping. Cardio improves your health, fitness level and has fat-burning benefits. Weight training can be cardiovascular if your exercises are performed in a consecutive circuit without breaks. In fact, I've included some high-rep and circuit-style workouts in this book that will increase your heart rate. However, in my experience, cardio is best handled as its own entity of fitness. Like the workouts in this book, a cardio workout doesn't require a gym membership. Walking, running, hiking and rollerblading are car-

dio activities that can be performed outdoors. If you want to work out in your home, try dancing, jumping rope and climbing up and down a flight of stairs. Of course, you can also do cardio on a piece of equipment, such as a treadmill or stairstepper. Enough with the lists—my point is that it's easy to incorporate cardiovascular exercise into your lifestyle. To get the benefits, include a 30-minute session at least three times a week. Up that frequency to four to five times a week if you're trying to lose weight. The workouts in this book are short enough to easily fit in before or after those sessions.

Resistance Training

Include weight training in your fitness routine at least twice a week. Even if your "weight" only consists of five-pound dumbbells, it's important to challenge your muscles with resistance. This type of training will strengthen and tone your muscles, and research shows it has important health implications as well. As we age, we lose bone density. Weight training can help your body preserve its bone density. This is especially important for women, whose bodies change dramatically following menopause. Strength training may also help fuel weight loss by increasing metabolism. Lastly, you'll look better if you can build more muscle.

Muscle takes up less space than fat, so a strong body often looks slimmer than a weak one. If you don't have much time, incorporate a strength-training routine into your program one or two times a week, doing one exercise for each part of your body. *Weights on the Ball Workbook* (Ulysses Press, 2004) is a great resource for resistance training at home, and makes a perfect companion to the workouts in this book.

Get Flexible

Stretching is another form of exercise, and it's important enough to be included in detail in this book. On the next page, you'll find recommendations for

TYPES OF STRETCHES

There are actually a few different types of stretches. For our purposes, we'll focus on the two most effective and common types: static and active. A *static stretch* is where you hold a muscle (or muscles) in a position. If you're seated with your legs extended out in front of you and you bend forward and hold the pose, that's a static stretch. An *active stretch* is where your muscle is forced to hold a contracted position, usually lifted or working against resistance. Standing and pulling one knee into your chest and holding it there is an active stretch.

how to include stretching in your program. Towards the end of the book, you'll find several stretches designed specifically for your core. While strengthening your core and performing cardio and resistance training is important, all would be for naught if you couldn't move your body. Include 5 to 10 minutes of stretching after every workout, being sure to perform a stretch for every part of your body worked in that session.

Duration

How long to hold a stretch is a point of contention among many health and fitness professionals. In yoga, stretches are sometimes held for several minutes; following a sports practice, many athletes hold stretches for 10 seconds. There is no definitive answer as to how long to hold a stretch, but 15 to 30 seconds seems to be the industry-supported norm and it's a good range for you to work with. I've found that this length of time is enough for my muscles to fully relax into a stretch.

Breathing

You should breathe deeply and with control when stretching. Never hold your breath! People often don't even realize they're holding their breath, so do a mental check of yourself as you stretch. It sometimes helps to recite "Inhale, Exhale" repeatedly in your head as you stretch. I find that this not only helps me control my breathing, the repetition aids in relaxation by forcing me to free my mind of all other thoughts and to focus only on letting go.

Stretching in Brief

It's difficult to summarize everything there is to know about stretching in a couple of pages. However, if you keep the following points in mind, you can safely start a stretching program.

Never stretch a cold muscle. You won't be as flexible and you could easily strain the muscle. Always perform a warm-up before you stretch, or stretch after a workout.

Stretch only to the point of mild tension. When you reach a point where you feel tightness, hold that position. If you feel like you can stretch farther once your muscles relax, carefully increase the stretch.

Stretching shouldn't be painful. If you experience pain during a stretch, release and try moving into it again. If you still feel pain, don't do the stretch. You may risk injury to a muscle or connective tissue.

Hold stretched positions, but never bounce. Bouncing can strain your muscles and cause injury.

The muscles on one side of your body are often more flexible than the other. Take this into account when doing side stretches and don't push a muscle beyond its limits. Be gentle on your body!

Make time for stretching after every workout. (Or even every day if your schedule permits.) Like any other healthy habit, stretching requires consistency and the benefits are greatest when you stretch your muscles regularly.

part two:

the
workouts

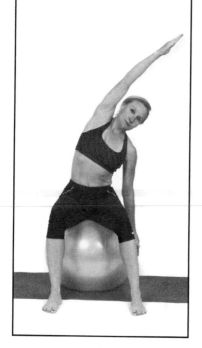

an overview

Your experience and goals are uniquely your own. The workouts in this section take that into account. Since they're multilevel, you can begin and progress at your own pace. What's more, there are also specialized workouts that allow you to target your training to the areas of your core you'd like to emphasize. Before you begin, read on to find out when to work out, how to warm up and cool down, and how to determine your current workout level.

When to Work Out

When's the best time to exercise? Some people say it's in the morning, before you've eaten, because the metabolism-revving effects of exercise will last throughout your day. Others say it's in the evening, after a day at work and before your evening meal. The answer is simple: The best time of day to exercise is whenever you're most likely to stick with it.

If you're not a morning person, don't try to compete with your natural clock and work out in the morning. You'll likely end up frustrated and resentful toward your workouts. Likewise, if you're exhausted at the end of your day, don't leave your workouts for the evening. You might use fatigue as an excuse to skip them. Listen to your biological clock and review your schedule to choose a time that works best for you. Then plan your exercise like you would any other important appointment and stick with it until it becomes a habit.

Level Yourself

Every workout has three levels: beginner, intermediate and advanced. (And in Part 3 you'll notice that each exercise has at least one variation based on the same three levels.) To figure out your current workout and exercise level, find the situation that best describes you in the chart on the next page and follow the recommendation. If you're not sure which level you're at, err on the side of caution and start out with the lower one. (You can always increase the intensity.)

Consistency Is Key

To get the best results, perform a core workout two to three times per week, resting at least 24 hours between workouts.

Now You're Getting Somewhere

As you progress, you'll need to increase the intensity of your

WORKOUT LEVEL CHART

I am...	You are at this workout level	You are at this exercise level
...a senior who doesn't exercise regularly	Beginner	Beginner
...someone who's never exercised	Beginner	Beginner
...returning to exercise after an injury	Beginner	Beginner/Intermediate
...returning to exercise after having a baby	Beginner	Beginner/Intermediate
...returning to exercise after being inactive for up to 8 weeks	Beginner	Intermediate
...a senior who exercises regularly	Intermediate	Beginner
...a beginner who has been doing the workouts in this book for six to eight weeks	Intermediate	Beginner/Intermediate
...someone who has exercised regularly for at least three months	Intermediate	Intermediate
...someone who has been doing the Intermediate level workouts, but no longer feels challenged	Advanced	Intermediate
...someone who has been exercising regularly for six months or longer	Advanced	Intermediate/Advanced
...someone who has been doing the Intermediate level workouts for six to eight weeks	Advanced	Advanced

workouts to continue seeing results and improvements. It's impossible to say when you'll be ready for the next level because you're an individual. However, after about six to eight weeks of working at the same level, you'll probably be ready to increase the challenge. Try moving on to the next level of workouts, but staying at the same exercise level. When you're feeling stronger, or are no longer seeing improvements, try the next level of the exercises. Please note that you might not ever get to the advanced level workouts and that's fine. (If you're a senior, you probably shouldn't since

your range of motion may be smaller than what's required.)

First Things First

Before performing any of the workouts that follow, warm up your body with at least 5 to 10 minutes of low-impact cardio. You can go for a walk, march in place, walk up and down a flight of stairs, or try this simple 5-minute warm-up:

1 March in place or do jumping jacks for 2 minutes.
2 Do Seated Hip Rolls (page 36) for 1 minute.
3 End with another 2 minutes of either marching in place or jumping jacks.

Cool It

Follow every workout with five minutes of stretching. Choose two to four stretches from the "Stretches on the Ball" section (page 128) and follow the instructions.

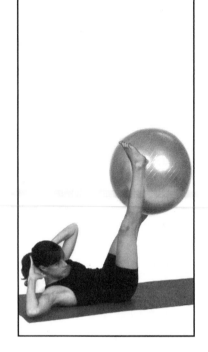

the workouts

The following workouts appear in this book. Be sure to follow the instructions for each workout as they're written, paying particular attention to the recommended order and rest.

Total Core Workouts

These workouts should form the foundation of your core training. Each is designed to take about 20–25 minutes to complete and effectively works every muscle of your core. Each level has two total core workouts. You can alternate between them, or perform one for several weeks and then switch to the other. Where a range is given for sets, begin with the minimum and only do the maximum if you feel strong enough.

5-Minute Total Core Blasts

Each of these workouts can be performed in about 5 minutes, depending on the speed of your reps and length of your rest periods. You can use these in either of two ways: as an extra challenge after your total core, cardio or other workout; or as a quick workout on its own. The latter removes the time excuse from your exercise equation— no matter how busy you are, you have 5 minutes in your day for fitness.

Elongating Workouts

Yoga and Pilates seem to elongate the muscles of practitioners. It's no wonder, since their exercises and poses often involve stretching your spine, which can help improve posture and thus make you stand taller. These workouts are inspired by movements found in the two practices. They work your entire core, so you can use them in place of one of your total core workouts once a week or whenever you need a change of pace.

Targeted Workouts

It's impossible to isolate one area of the abdominals or back when you're exercising. However, there are many exercises that emphasize one area over another. (Moving your torso from side to side, for example, more heavily targets the obliques.) The targeted workouts are designed to emphasize different parts of your core: your lower abs, upper abs, obliques (sides of your waist) and back. Each workout will take about 10–15 minutes to perform, depending on how quickly you move through your reps and how long you rest. You can use these workouts once a week instead of a total core workout to work on a specific area.

total core workouts

workout 1

BEGINNER TOTAL CORE

	PAGE	EXERCISE	SETS	REPS
	36	seated hip roll	2–3	5
	54	rollback	2–3	5
	44	rotating knee raise	2–3	5
	72	back extension	2–3	5

INSTRUCTIONS: Do 1 set of each exercise in the order listed. Then repeat the rotation, beginning with the first exercise. Rest for 1 minute between each set.

workout 2

BEGINNER TOTAL CORE

	PAGE	EXERCISE	SETS	REPS
	106	crunch with feet on ball	2–3	5
	114	bridge	2–3	5
	42	side-to-side reach	2–3	5
	84	around the world	2–3	5

INSTRUCTIONS: Do 1 set of each exercise in the order listed. Then repeat the rotation, beginning with the first exercise. Rest for 1 minute between each set

workout 1

INTERMEDIATE TOTAL CORE

	PAGE	EXERCISE	SETS	REPS
	50	ball crunch	3	10
	58	reverse plank	3	hold for 30–60 sec
	108	oblique crunch with feet on ball	3	10
	102	leg crosses	3	10

INSTRUCTIONS: Perform 1 set of each exercise in the order listed, resting for 30 seconds between each set. Repeat the rotation twice more, beginning with the first exercise each time.

workout 2

INTERMEDIATE TOTAL CORE

	PAGE	EXERCISE	SETS	REPS
	96	straight-body crunch	3	10
	110	reverse crunch	3	10
	116	lying leg rotation	3	10
	68	swimming kicks	3	10

INSTRUCTIONS: Perform 1 set of each exercise in the order listed, resting for 30 seconds between each set. Repeat the rotation twice more, beginning with the first exercise each time.

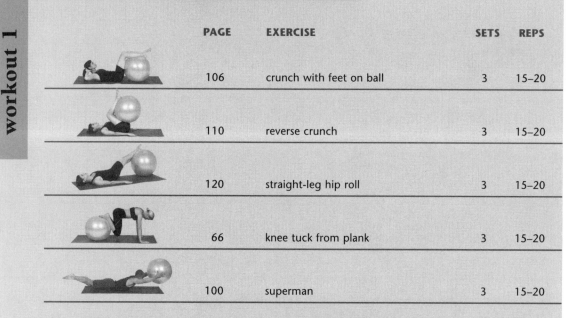

workout 1

ADVANCED TOTAL CORE

	PAGE	EXERCISE	SETS	REPS
	106	crunch with feet on ball	3	15–20
	110	reverse crunch	3	15–20
	120	straight-leg hip roll	3	15–20
	66	knee tuck from plank	3	15–20
	100	superman	3	15–20

INSTRUCTIONS: Perform 1 set of each exercise in the order listed, moving from one exercise to the next without rest. After completing 1 rotation of the exercises, rest for 1 to 2 minutes before starting over again. Repeat.

workout 2

ADVANCED TOTAL CORE

	PAGE	EXERCISE	SETS	REPS
	124	double-leg stretch	3	15–20
	118	legs overhead	3	15–20
	64	plank twist	3	15–20
	122	lying straight-leg lifts	3	15–20
	72	back extension	3	15–20

INSTRUCTIONS: Perform 1 set of each exercise in the order listed, moving from one exercise to the next without rest. After completing 1 rotation of the exercises, rest for 1 to 2 minutes before starting over again. Repeat.

5-minute total core blasts

BEGINNER

	106	crunch with feet on ball	1–2	5
	40	side twist	1–2	5
	86	straight-leg deadlift	1–2	5

INSTRUCTIONS: Perform the exercises in the order listed, doing 1 set of each exercise and resting for 30 seconds between each set. If you choose to, begin with the first exercise and repeat.

INTERMEDIATE

	50	ball crunch	2	10
	102	leg crosses	2	10
	76	side leg lift	2	10

INSTRUCTIONS: Perform 1 set of each exercise in the order listed, resting for 30 seconds between each set. Repeat.

ADVANCED

	66	knee tuck from plank	2	15–20
	52	oblique ball crunch	2	15–20
	110	reverse crunch	2	15–20

INSTRUCTIONS: Perform the exercises in the order listed, moving from one exercise to the next without rest. When you've completed 1 rotation of the exercises, rest for 1 minute and then repeat.

elongating workouts

BEGINNER					
		94	roll-up	2	5
		78	roll-out	2	5
		80	kneeling rotation	2	5

INSTRUCTIONS: Do 1 set of each exercise in the order listed, resting for 1 minute between each set. Then repeat the rotation, beginning with the first exercise.

INTERMEDIATE					
		62	plank	3	hold for 30–60 sec
		92	scissors	3	10
		118	legs overhead	3	10
		70	opposition raise	3	10

INSTRUCTIONS: Perform 1 set of each exercise in the order listed, resting for 30 seconds between each set. Repeat the rotation twice more, beginning with the first exercise each time.

ADVANCED					
		124	double-leg stretch	3	15
		122	lying straight-leg lifts	3	15
		94	roll-up	3	15
		88	seated straddle twist	3	15

INSTRUCTIONS: Perform 1 set of each exercise in the order listed, moving from one exercise to the next without rest. After completing 1 rotation of the exercises, rest for 1 to 2 minutes before starting over again. Repeat.

elongating

targeted workouts: lower abs

BEGINNER				
	38	knee raise	2	5
	110	reverse crunch	2	5
	92	scissors	2	5

INSTRUCTIONS: Perform the exercises in the order listed, resting for one minute between each set. Repeat.

INTERMEDIATE				
	44	rotating knee raise	3	10
	110	reverse crunch	3	10
	122	lying straight-leg lifts	3	10

INSTRUCTIONS: Perform 1 set of each exercise in the order listed, resting for 30 seconds between each set. Repeat the rotation twice more, beginning with the first exercise each time.

ADVANCED				
	110	reverse crunch	3	15–20
	66	knee tuck from plank	3	15–20
	112	reverse crunch twist	3	15–20
	102	leg crosses	3	15–20

INSTRUCTIONS: Perform the exercises in the order listed, moving from one exercise to the next without rest. After completing 1 set of each exercise, rest for 1 minute and then begin the rotation again.

targeted

targeted workouts: upper abs

BEGINNER

106	crunch with feet on ball	2	5
96	straight-body crunch	2	5
118	legs overhead	2	5

INSTRUCTIONS: Do 1 set of each exercise in the order listed. Then repeat the rotation, beginning with the first exercise. Rest for 1 minute between each set.

INTERMEDIATE

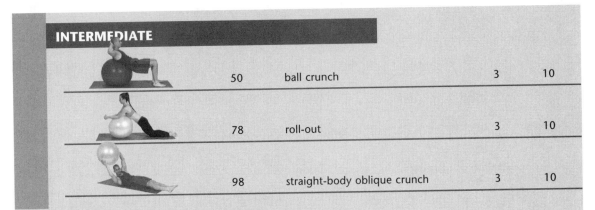

50	ball crunch	3	10
78	roll-out	3	10
98	straight-body oblique crunch	3	10

INSTRUCTIONS: Perform 1 set of each exercise in the order listed, resting for 30 seconds between each set. Repeat the rotation twice more, beginning with the first exercise each time.

ADVANCED

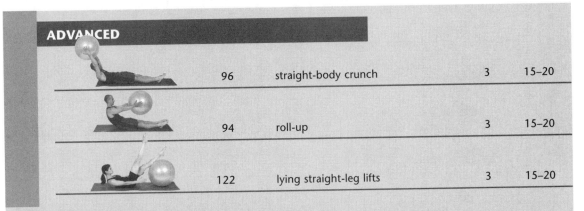

96	straight-body crunch	3	15–20
94	roll-up	3	15–20
122	lying straight-leg lifts	3	15–20

INSTRUCTIONS: Perform all sets of the first exercise, resting 30 seconds between each set, before moving on to the second exercise. Repeat with the second and third exercises.

targeted workouts: obliques

BEGINNER

Page	Exercise	Sets	Reps
40	side twist	2	5
42	side-to-side reach	2	5
80	kneeling rotation	2	5

INSTRUCTIONS: Do 1 set of each exercise, resting for 1 minute between each set. Then repeat the exercises.

INTERMEDIATE

Page	Exercise	Sets	Reps
52	oblique ball crunch	3	10
56	reclined rotation	3	10
64	plank twist	3	10
82	side crunch	3	10

INSTRUCTIONS: Perform 1 set of each exercise in the order listed, resting for 30 seconds between each set. Repeat the rotation twice more, beginning with the first exercise each time.

ADVANCED

Page	Exercise	Sets	Reps
98	straight-body oblique crunch	3	15–20
126	straight-leg bicycles	3	15–20
120	straight-leg hip roll	3	15–20
116	lying leg rotation	3	15–20
44	rotating knee raise	3	15–20

INSTRUCTIONS: Perform the exercises in the order listed, moving from one exercise to the next without rest. After completing 1 set of each exercise, rest for 1 minute and then begin the rotation again.

targeted

targeted workouts: back

BEGINNER

72	back extension	2	5
48	flye to pullover	2	5
84	around the world	2	5

INSTRUCTIONS: Do 1 set of each exercise in the order listed. Then repeat the rotation, beginning with the first exercise. Rest for 1 minute between each set.

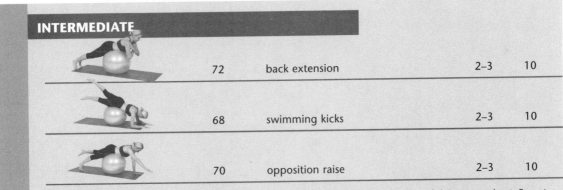

INTERMEDIATE

72	back extension	2–3	10
68	swimming kicks	2–3	10
70	opposition raise	2–3	10

INSTRUCTIONS: Perform 1 set of each exercise in the order listed, resting for 30 seconds between each set. Repeat the rotation once or twice more, beginning with the first exercise each time.

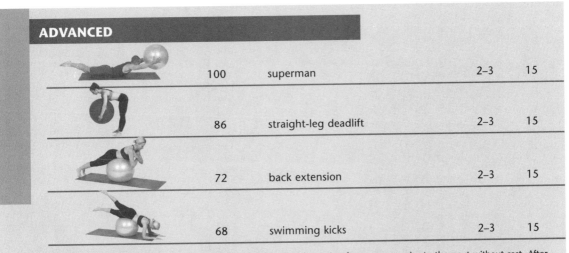

ADVANCED

100	superman	2–3	15
86	straight-leg deadlift	2–3	15
72	back extension	2–3	15
68	swimming kicks	2–3	15

INSTRUCTIONS: Perform the exercises in the order listed, moving from one exercise to the next without rest. After completing 1 set of each exercise, rest for 1 minute and then begin the rotation again.

targeted

part three:
the exercises

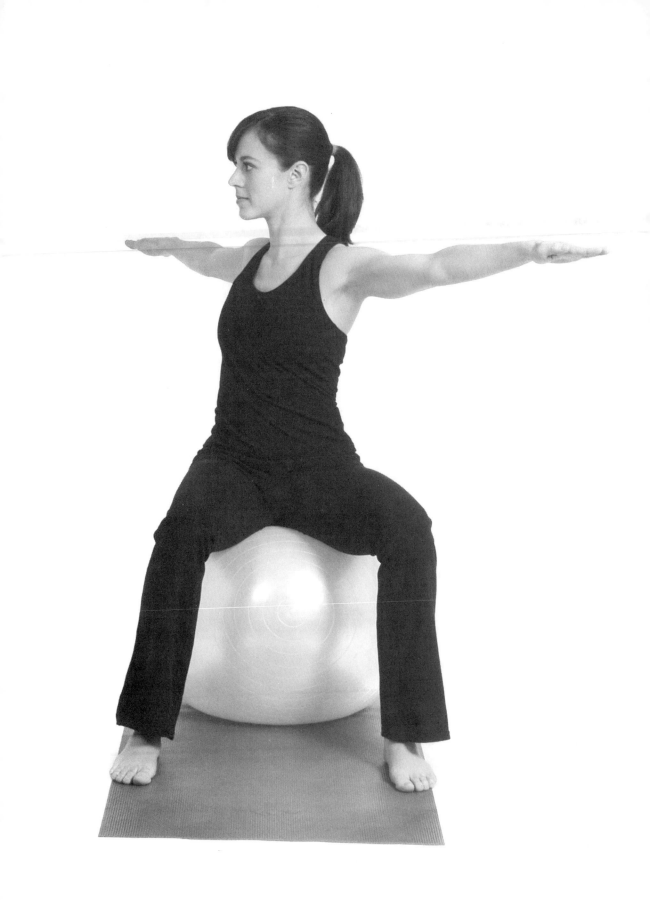

sitting on the ball

Sitting on the ball forces all the muscles of your core to engage to stabilize your position. That means even if you just sit still, you're working your abs and back. These exercises not only challenge your core, they can also improve your posture, as it's difficult to balance on a spherical surface if you're not sitting upright. When you're set up properly (seated "upright"), your head, neck and shoulders should be aligned. To maintain this alignment, imagine a string pulling you up from the top of your head.

seated hip roll

This is a good warm-up for your entire core. It's also a great way to relax your back muscles after a long period spent seated.

STARTING POSITION: Sit on the ball, bending your knees 90 degrees and placing your feet, hip-width apart, flat on the floor. Contract your abs to put your spine in a neutral position and raise your arms out to your sides into a T. Take a moment to stabilize your position on the ball. **INHALE** to begin.

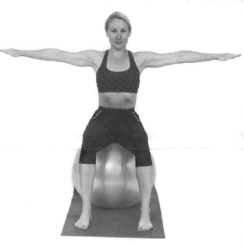

1

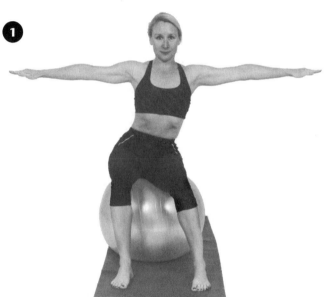

1 As you **EXHALE**, roll your pelvis to the right, moving the ball slightly to the right.

variations

INTERMEDIATE

Roll your hips in a smooth, circular motion. Begin by rolling in one direction, then switch to the other. Think of a hula dancer: The movement should be fluid, not choppy, stopping only to switch directions.

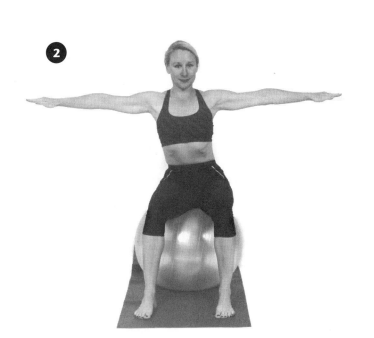

2

2 INHALE to return to center. **EXHALE** and roll your hips to the left, moving the ball slightly to the left.

Return to the starting position.

INTERMEDIATE/ADVANCED

Move your hips forward and back and add your arms and legs. As you **INHALE**, shift your hips back as you straighten your legs and extend your arms straight out in front of you at chest height. (Your feet will be flexed and your legs will be nearly straight in this position.) As you **EXHALE**, push your hips forward, returning your legs to their bent starting position, and pull your arms back to a T.

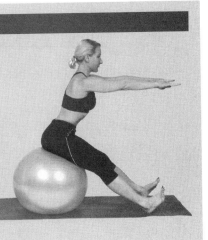

knee raise

This exercise is deceptively simple. The slight movement of raising your leg while balancing on the ball takes great effort on the part of your lower abs.

STARTING POSITION: Sit on the ball, bending your knees 90 degrees and placing your feet, hip-width apart, flat on the floor. Draw your shoulder blades up then back and down. Tighten your abs to support your seated position. Raise your arms straight out to your sides into a T. **INHALE** to begin.

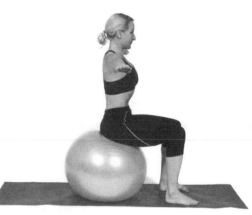

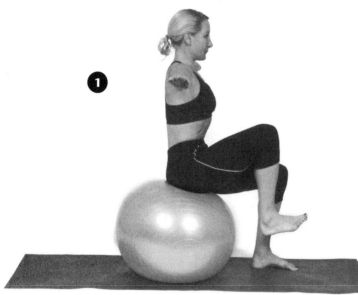

1 As you **EXHALE**, lift your right knee toward your chest, keeping your leg bent and torso upright.

variations

BEGINNING

Keep your arms at the sides of the ball for support. You may also put the ball against a wall for additional support.

INTERMEDIATE

Instead of bending your knee and raising it toward your chest, straighten your leg and extend it out in front of you. Lift and lower the leg then switch sides and repeat.

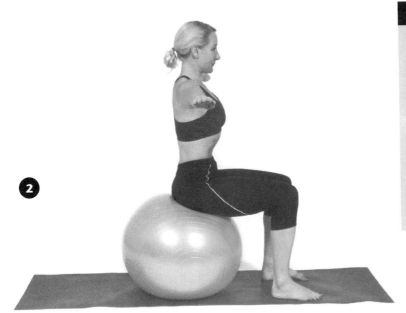

2

TIPS

- Your upper body remains still throughout the exercise; only your legs move.
- If you feel yourself bending forward as you raise your knee, you're raising it too high.
- Focus on a stable point in front of you. This will help you balance on the ball, and also prevent you from leaning into your knee.

2 **INHALE** as you lower your right leg back to the starting position. Switch sides and repeat.

ADVANCED

Perform the intermediate version, but raise your arms straight overhead. Keep them raised for all reps.

side twist

Rotating your torso while keeping your lower body steady works the sides of your waist. The movement also stretches the muscles that support your spine.

STARTING POSITION: Sit on the ball with your knees just wider than your hips. Bend your knees 90 degrees and place your feet flat on the floor. Contract your abs to stabilize your position on the ball and support your back. Raise your arms straight out to your sides into a T. **INHALE** to begin.

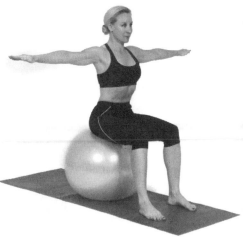

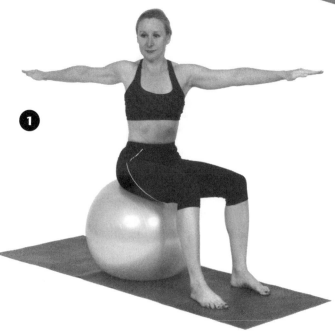

1

1 As you **EXHALE**, slowly twist to the right as far as you comfortably can, leading with your shoulders instead of your head. Your head should remain aligned with your neck throughout the movement.

variations

BEGINNING

Instead of raising your arms, place your palms on the sides of the ball. As you rotate to your right, allow your left hand to brush along the ball and your left knee as your right hand moves toward the back of the ball.

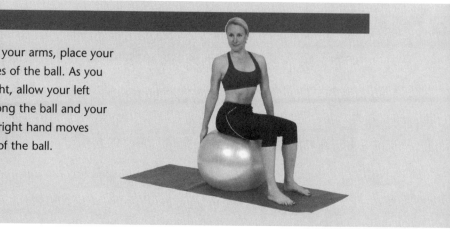

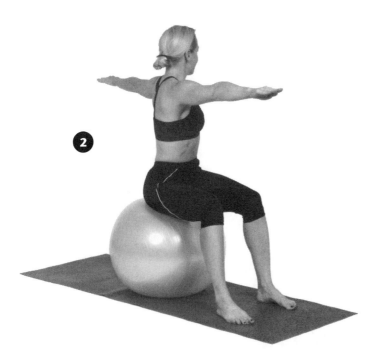

2

- Your hips should not move in this exercise: Think of your hipbones as headlights and keep them facing forward.
- If you feel your hips move, you're rotating beyond your range of motion. Decrease the amount of your twist.
- If your lower back feels stiff, slow down the movement.
- Move your body with your breath. As you become more flexible, you might move more quickly from side to side.

2 **INHALE** to return to center. **EXHALE** and twist as far as you can to the left.

Return to the starting position.

ADVANCED

With a flat back, bend forward at your waist so that your chest nearly touches your knees. Extend your arms out to your sides and slowly twist to the right so that you face the right side of the room and your arms make a diagonal line from floor to ceiling. Return to center and twist to the opposite side.

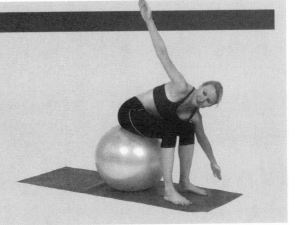

side-to-side reach

This exercise effectively targets your obliques—the muscles at the sides of your waist.

STARTING POSITION: Sit on the ball, bending your knees and placing your feet flat on the floor, hip-width apart. Rest your arms alongside your body, with your palms touching—not clutching—the ball. **INHALE** to begin.

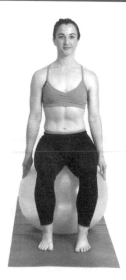

1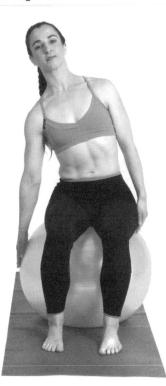

1 As you **EXHALE**, reach the fingertips of your right hand toward the floor on the right side of your body. Only bend the upper half of your torso; your lower body remains still and your hips remain squared.

INTERMEDIATE

Place your hands, fingers unclasped, behind your head. Bend sideways from your waist toward one side, lowering your elbow toward the ball. Return to center and repeat on the opposite side.

variations

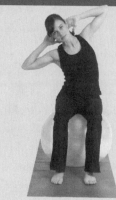

TIPS

• Reach your hand—don't just lower it—toward the floor to help you get a stronger contraction out of the obliques.

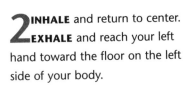

2 **INHALE** and return to center. **EXHALE** and reach your left hand toward the floor on the left side of your body.

Return to the starting position.

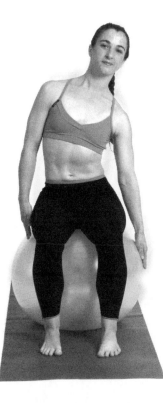

ADVANCED

Place your hands, fingers unclasped, behind your head. As you bend sideways, slightly push your hips toward the opposite side as your elbow reaches down. This will increase the degree of the reach.

rotating knee raise

Balancing on one leg when your feet are spread wide increases the difficulty by making it harder to stabilize your body. Adding the twist puts the obliques and spine extensors to work.

STARTING POSITION: Sit on the ball, legs bent and spread wider than your hips, feet flat on the floor. Stack your torso so that your body forms a straight line from your head to your hips. Raise your arms straight out to your sides into a T, palms down. **INHALE** to begin.

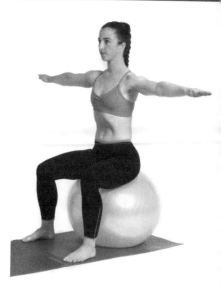

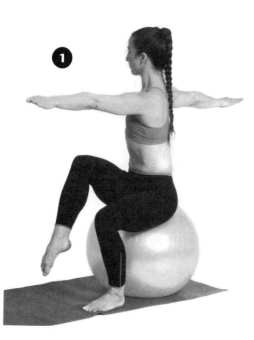

1 As you **EXHALE**, lift your right knee as you rotate your torso toward the right side of the room. Remain upright even as you twist—don't bend forward. Keep your non-lifting leg completely still.

variations

BEGINNING

Place your legs hip-width apart, feet flat on the floor. Moving your legs closer together makes it easier to stabilize your body as you lift your opposing leg.

INTERMEDIATE

Place your hands, fingers unclasped, behind your head, then perform the exercise. This prevents you from using your arms to help you balance and forces your core to work harder to stabilize your position.

2

2 **INHALE** as you slowly lower your leg—being careful to maintain the wide-leg stance—and return your torso to center.

3

3 **EXHALE** and lift your left knee as you rotate your torso toward the left side of the room.

Return to the starting position.

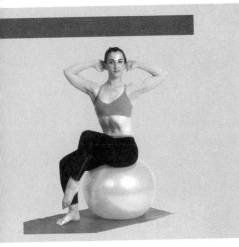

ADVANCED

To further increase the challenge, do this exercise with 2- to 3-pound ankle weights. The added resistance increases the workload on your abs.

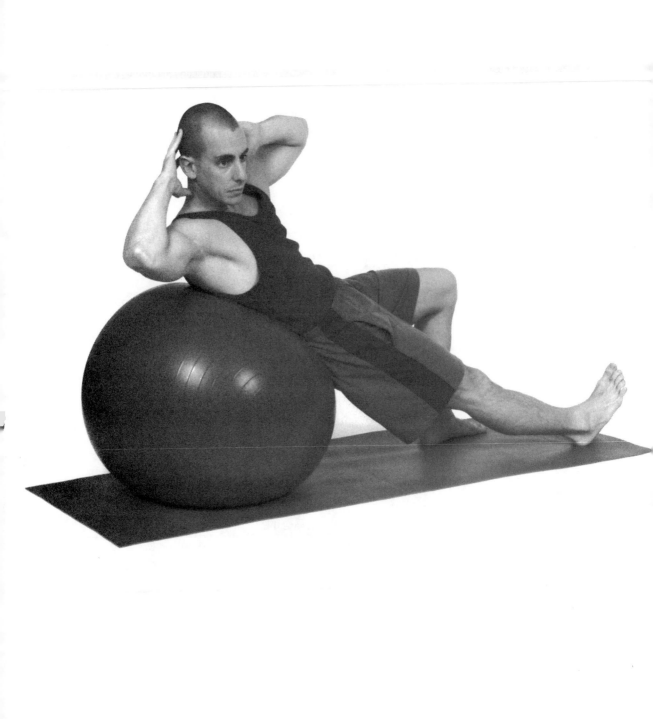

back on the ball

Although the back-on-the ball position may seem basic, you'll find that its benefits extend way beyond your core. When you perform exercises with your back against the ball instead of the floor, you work the muscles of your midsection through a fuller range of motion. What's more, this position simultaneously engages many of your larger muscle groups, including legs and chest, to stabilize and support your body as it moves. Think of these exercises as total-body strengtheners with an emphasis on the core.

flye to pullover

Although you work your back and chest muscles in this exercise, you'll feel your abs elongate and contract as you reach your arms around your body.

STARTING POSITION: Sit on the ball and walk your feet out until only your upper back and neck are supported by the ball. Place your feet flat on the floor, legs slightly wider than hip-width apart and bent to form right angles. Lift your pelvis slightly so that your body forms a straight line from your knees to your head. Keep your body elongated throughout the exercise. Contract your abs and extend your arms out from your chest so that they're perpendicular to the ceiling and your palms are facing in. **INHALE** to begin.

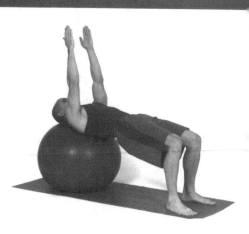

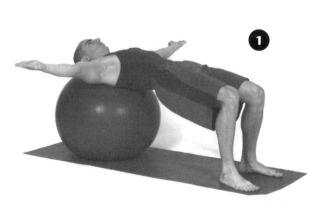

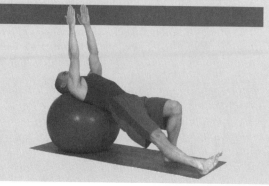

1 As you **EXHALE**, open your chest and extend your arms out your sides until your upper arms are parallel to the floor.

2 **INHALE** and, pulling from your chest, raise your arms back to the starting position.

INTERMEDIATE

Straighten one leg, extending it in front of you, foot flexed and heel on the floor. Keep it extended for all reps of one set, then switch legs for the next set.

variations

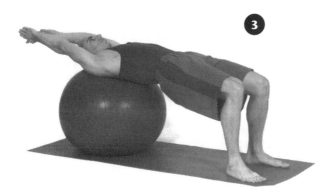

3

3 EXHALE as you slowly stretch your arms overhead in an arc-like motion, elongating your back. Only stretch to the point of mild tension; don't stretch so far that your back arches.

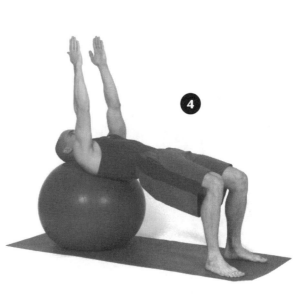

4

4 INHALE as you use your upper back and chest to pull your arms up to the starting position.

ADVANCED

Perform the exercise with both legs extended straight out in front of you, feet either pointed or flexed. This makes it harder to balance, which increases the challenge on the core.

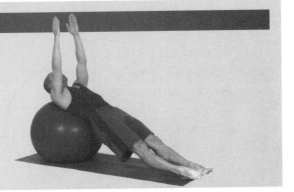

ball crunch

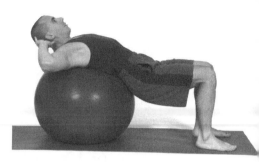

Performing the crunch on the ball works your rectus abdominis through a full range of motion. The distance between where you start and finish is small, so you only need to lift your shoulder blades off the ball.

STARTING POSITION: Sit on the ball. Slowly walk your feet forward, letting the ball roll back until your entire torso—from shoulder blades to hips—is supported by the ball. Place your feet flat on the floor, hip-width apart, and bend your knees 90 degrees. Put your hands, fingers unclasped, behind your head. Take a moment to stabilize your position on the ball, ensuring it will not roll out from beneath you. **INHALE** to begin.

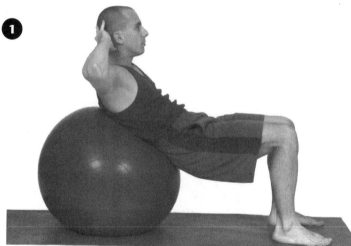

1 **EXHALE** and, keeping your neck neutral, tighten your abs as you slowly curl your torso upward. You should feel a contraction in your abs.

variations

INTERMEDIATE

Stretch your arms overhead so that your biceps are next to your ears. Clasp one hand with the other. Keep your arms in this outstretched position throughout the movement, being careful not to duck your head forward as you lift.

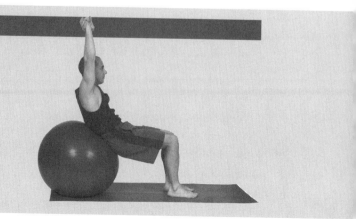

2 **INHALE** and, keeping your abs tight, slowly lower your body to the starting position.

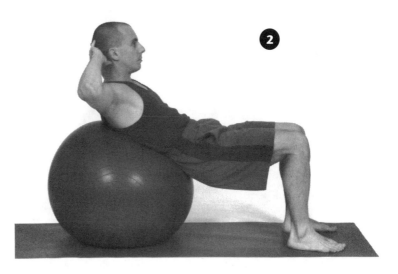

ADVANCED

From the main starting position, walk your feet farther forward until only the uppermost part of your torso—your upper back and shoulder blades—is supported by the ball. Perform the crunch from this position.

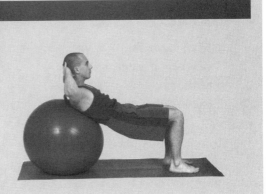

oblique ball crunch

This crunch is actually two parts performed in a flowing motion on one exhale: lift to the center and twist to the opposite side.

STARTING POSITION: Sit on the ball. Slowly walk your feet forward, letting the ball roll back until your entire torso—from shoulder blades to hips—is supported by the ball. Place your feet flat on the floor, hip-width apart, and bend your knees 90 degrees. Put your hands, fingers unclasped, behind your head. Take a moment to stabilize your position on the ball, ensuring it will not roll out from beneath you. Contract your abs to bring your spine to a neutral position. **INHALE** to begin.

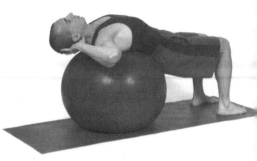

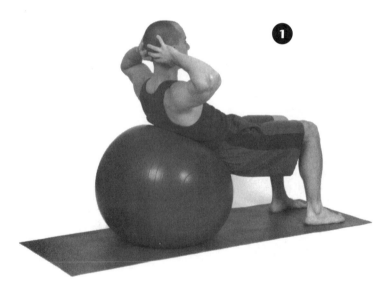

1 As you **EXHALE**, raise your shoulder blades off the ball, being careful not to pull on your neck.

INTERMEDIATE

Straighten the leg you are crunching toward. This makes it harder to stabilize your position on the ball.

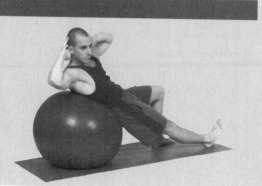

variations

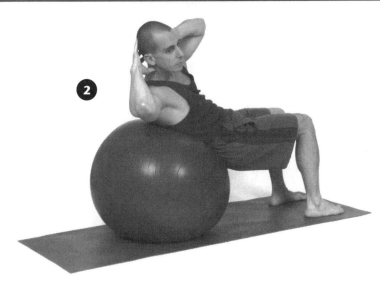

TIPS

- Concentrate on twisting your shoulder, not your elbow.
- Put your opposite hand on the side you're bending toward (e.g., place your left hand on your left side as you crunch your right elbow to your left knee) so that you can feel the obliques working.

2 Continuing to **EXHALE**, twist your left shoulder toward your right thigh. Don't rush the movement or force the twist. Breathe slowly and deliberately and use your breath to guide your movement.

3 **INHALE** as you reverse the movement and lower to the starting position. Repeat to the left side.

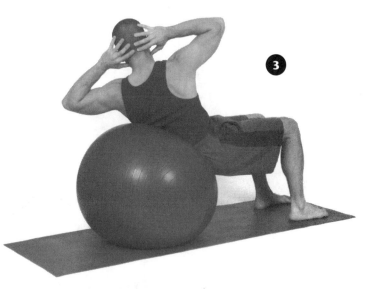

ADVANCED

Bring your opposite knee up toward the opposite shoulder as you crunch. This increases the intensity of the movement on your abs.

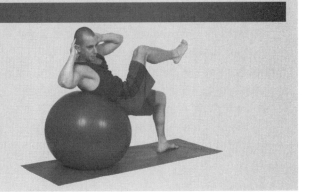

rollback

By eliminating your arms from the movement of rolling back, your abs and back must engage to keep your body balanced. What's more, you'll need to roll back slowly and with control, which means your muscles will stay engaged longer than during a movement performed at a quicker pace.

STARTING POSITION: Sit on the ball, as far forward as you can while still balancing. (Only your butt is supported by the ball.) Your knees are bent and feet are flat on the floor, hip-width apart. Roll your shoulders down your back and together. Your entire upper body—from head and neck to shoulders and hips—should be aligned. Cross your arms in front of your chest.

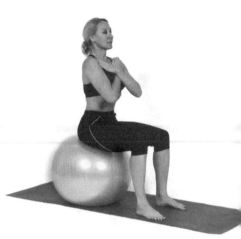

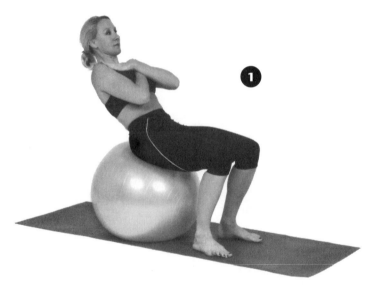

1 INHALE as you contract your abs and tilt your hips slightly forward. Maintain the pelvic tilt throughout the movement. This will keep your spine in its naturally rounded position and ensure that the abs, not your hip flexors, do the work. **EXHALE** and slowly roll backward on the ball.

INTERMEDIATE

Extend your arms overhead. As you roll back, bring them out to your sides. At the end of the movement, when you're lying on the ball, reach your arms straight out in front of you.

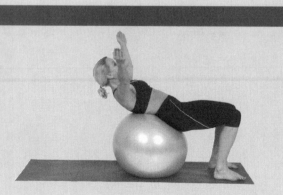

variations

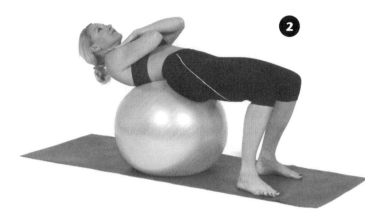

2

2 Continue rolling backward until the middle of your back makes contact with the ball. **INHALE**.

3 Keeping your abs contracted, **EXHALE** and curl your chest toward your hips as you roll up to the starting position. Make sure you return all the way to the upright, seated position. Restack your body—head, neck, shoulders and pelvis aligned—before rolling back again.

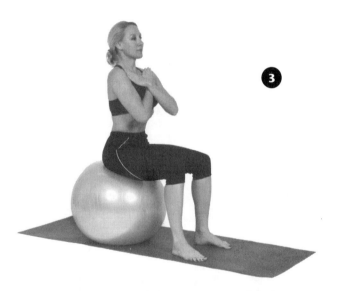

3

ADVANCED

Hold a dumbbell with both hands at your chest. The added resistance increases the workload on your abs.

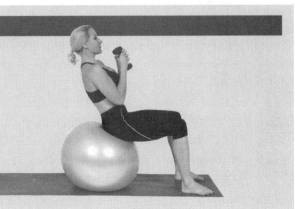

reclined rotation

The rotation here has the added benefit of limbering the ligaments of your lower back.

STARTING POSITION: Sit on the ball with your feet flat on the floor, legs slightly wider than hip-width apart. Slowly walk your feet forward and roll back until your entire back is supported by the ball. Extend your arms straight out from your chest, palms facing in and fingers pointing toward the ceiling. Slightly lift your head so that it is aligned with your shoulders. Contract your abs to put your spine in a neutral position. Keeping your lower body completely still, **INHALE**.

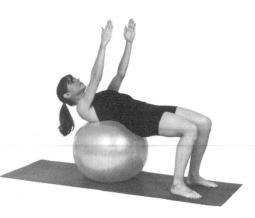

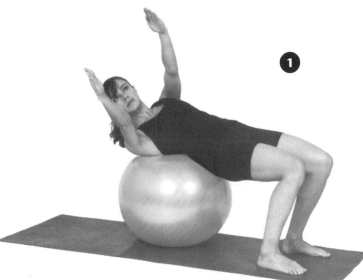

1

1 As you **EXHALE**, turn your torso toward your right side (both arms will turn as well; your bottom arm should move through a 90-degree turn). Your left hip will rise slightly and the ball will roll slightly to the left, but try to keep your butt pressed against the ball. Keep your lower body still by contracting your abs as much as possible.

variations

BEGINNING

Perform this exercise with the ball positioned against a wall and your legs spread wider apart. These changes make it easier to stabilize your position. If this is still too challenging, perform this exercise on the floor. Lie on the floor with your knees bent and feet flat on the floor. Extend your arms straight out from your chest and twist from side to side.

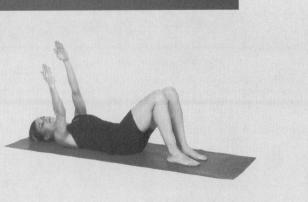

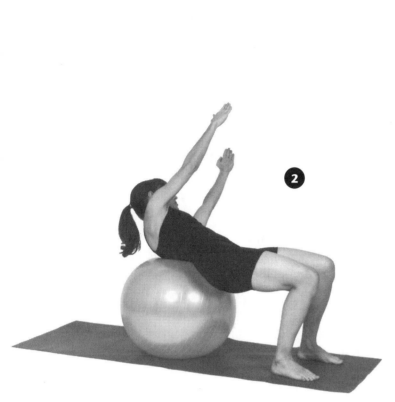

2

TIPS

- To increase the twist, think about reaching your bottom hand toward the floor.
- Only your upper body rotates. Keep your lower body grounded throughout the exercise by pressing through your heels.

2 INHALE as you return to center and repeat to the left.

Return to the starting position.

ADVANCED

Hold a dumbbell with both hands and extend your arms straight out from your chest. Twist from side to side, being careful to maintain control and not let the weight of the dumbbell pull you.

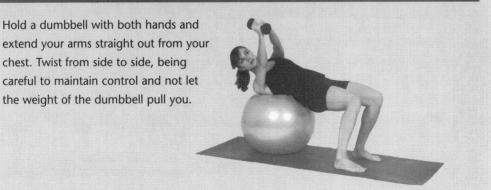

reverse plank

Balancing your body in unusual positions—like this exercise—improves your control. Squeezing your butt will help you maintain the position. The buttocks muscles are also great assistors in the intermediate or advanced variations.

STARTING POSITION: Sit on the floor with the ball placed in front of you. Place your hands, palms down and fingers facing forward, at your sides about a foot behind you. Place your legs on top of the ball, pushing it forward until your calves are resting on the ball and your body forms a V. **INHALE** to begin.

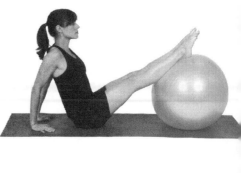

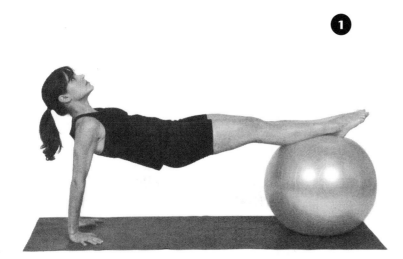

1 As you **EXHALE**, lift your hips until your body is in a plank position, with knees, hips and torso forming a straight line. Your legs are straight and pressed together; point your toes to activate your leg muscles. Your shoulders are aligned with your wrists and your head is slightly raised. Contract your abs to prevent your belly from sagging. Hold the position for three full breaths.

INTERMEDIATE

Add movement to this stability exercise by lowering your hips toward the floor on your second exhale, then lifting them back up. Don't allow your butt to touch the floor as you lower.

variations

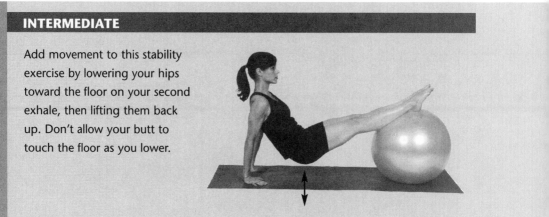

- Imagine your fingers as roots of a tree. Spread them out and press them into the floor to ground your arms and take some pressure off your wrists.
- Make sure your belly isn't sagging or pushing out. Either mistake will put pressure on your lower back.
- Think about extending out through the top and bottom of your body.

2 Lower yourself to the floor, keeping your legs on the ball, and have a seat. Relax your hands before beginning the next rep.

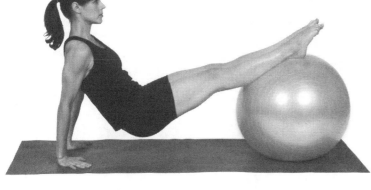

ADVANCED

Do the intermediate movement and lean forward as you lower your hips to "crunch" your body in half.

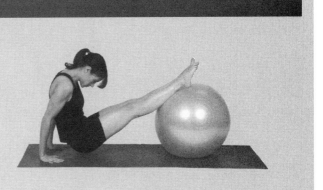

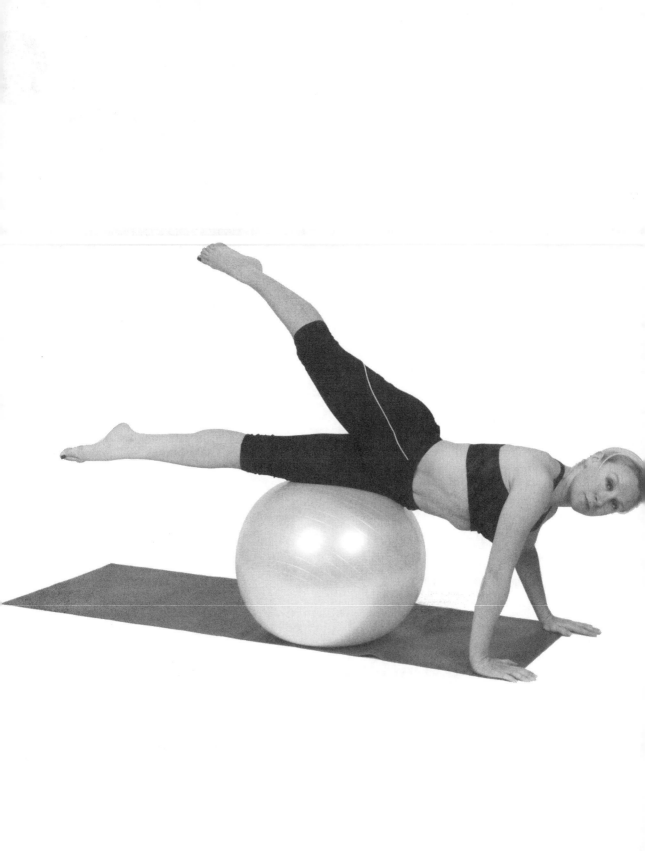

lying face down on the ball

Exercises that are performed face down on the ball are super-effective for your core—your abs and back must engage to keep you stabilized in this position. These moves also help improve your posture since it's challenging to keep your spine in a natural position while your arms or legs move. Whether you're holding still in Plank or moving in a Back Extension, working your core while face down provides a good balance to exercises performed on your back.

plank

Although all of your core muscles are recruited to stabilize your position, your transverse abdominis is worked particularly hard. If you're doing this for the first time, try it in front of a mirror, or have a friend check your alignment, to make sure your positioning is correct.

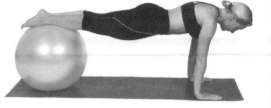

STARTING POSITION: From a kneeling position, drape your body over the ball. Place your palms flat on the floor in front of you and extend your legs straight out behind you. Slowly walk your hands forward until the ball is beneath your shins. Keep your legs together and point your toes. Align your shoulders with your wrists and spread your fingers wide apart.

variations

BEGINNING

Only roll out to the point where your hips are supported by the ball. This will make it easier to stabilize your position.

1 INHALE and contract your abs to create a flat surface and remove the arch from your back. Your entire body should form a straight line in the plank position. Keep your head aligned with your shoulders and stare down at the floor beneath you. Extend out through the top of your head and the bottoms of your feet. **EXHALE** and **INHALE** for three to five breaths, holding your body still.

TIPS

- If your belly sags, you're not using your core. Imagine someone pulling you up from your lower back and hold that position for all breaths.
- Make sure your shoulders don't jut forward or behind your wrists. This will strain your wrists.
- Imagine one string pulling you from your head while another pulls you from your toes.

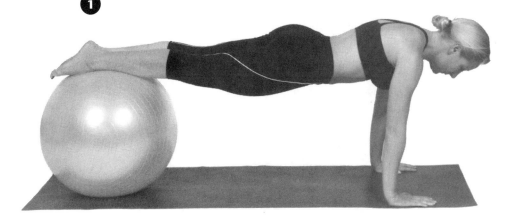

ADVANCED

Walk your hands out until only the tops of your feet are supported by the ball. When less of your body is supported on the ball, it's harder to maintain your balance.

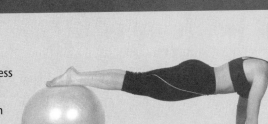

plank twist

This is an effective move for trimming the sides of your waists, and your arms will get a workout as well.

STARTING POSITION: Drape your body over the ball and place your palms flat on the floor. Slowly walk your hands forward until the ball is beneath your hips and lower abdominals, and your body forms a straight line from your head to your feet. Align your wrists beneath your shoulders; keep your head aligned with your neck. Contract your abs to put your spine in a neutral position. **INHALE** to begin.

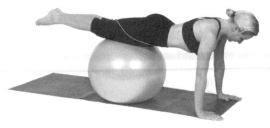

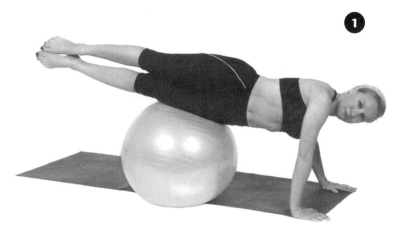

1

1 As you **EXHALE**, twist your hips to the right, allowing the ball to roll beneath you. Continue twisting until your hips are turned 90 degrees to your shoulders. Your opposite arm will bend slightly as you twist. The movement is controlled, but not slow.

variations

BEGINNING

Drape your upper body over the ball and extend your legs straight behind you, with your toes tucked under and touching the floor. Your chest is supported by the ball and your elbows are right in front of it, hands on the floor.

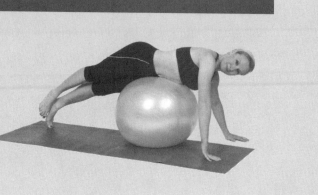

2 Once you reach the point where your hips are at a right angle to your shoulders, **INHALE** and immediately begin twisting back to the starting position. Repeat on the other side.

2

ADVANCED

When you twist, open and split your legs so that the top leg reaches up and back while the lower leg pulls forward.

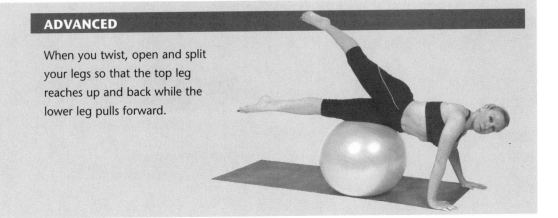

knee tuck from plank

Adding the knee tuck makes the plank a movement exercise, and has the added bonus of working your legs, arms and shoulders as well as your core. This is an intermediate movement.

STARTING POSITION: Lie face down on the ball with your palms flat on the floor. Carefully walk your arms forward until just your shins and the tops of your feet are on top of the ball. To protect your neck, keep your head aligned and look straight down at the space between your hands. Your body should form a straight line from your head to your feet. Your wrists are in line with your shoulders, and should remain so for the entire movement. **INHALE** to begin.

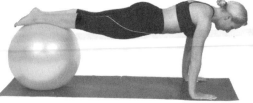

1

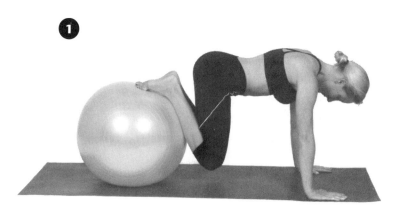

1 EXHALE and, contracting your abs, pull your knees in toward your chest, keeping your upper body in the starting position. The ball will roll toward you, but you should be in control of its movement.

variations

BEGINNING

If you are just starting out, do not attempt the tuck. Instead, hold your body in the supported plank position, with your shins on the ball, for 30 seconds.

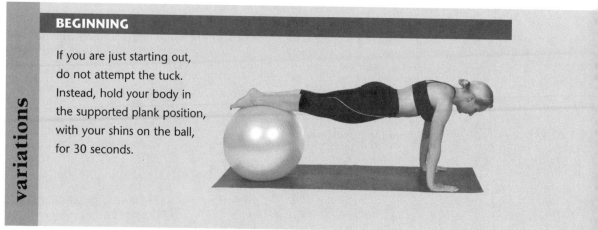

TIPS

- If your lower back feels strained, do the beginner variation.
- Don't drop your chin onto your chest. Keep your head, neck and shoulders aligned throughout the movement.

2 **INHALE** and, slowly and with control, straighten your legs to the starting position.

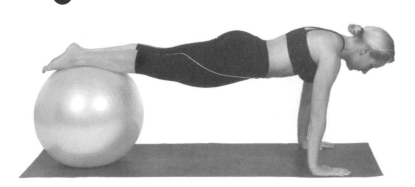

ADVANCED

As your knees tuck in, curl your chest in to meet them. This increases the challenge to your core.

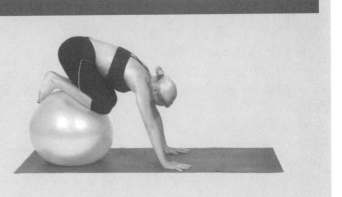

swimming kicks

Keeping your legs straight as you raise and lower them takes the emphasis away from your glutes and puts it on your lower back.

STARTING POSITION: Kneel behind the ball and drape your body over it. Roll forward until your torso is supported by the ball. Extend your legs straight out behind you, toes pointed and tops of feet pressed into floor. Place your forearms on the floor in front of the ball, palms down and fingers pointing forward. Lean forward onto your forearms, allowing your head to naturally fall, until your legs are raised off the floor and your body is aligned diagonally from head to toes. Contract your abs to put your spine in a neutral position and to protect your back as you kick. **INHALE** to begin.

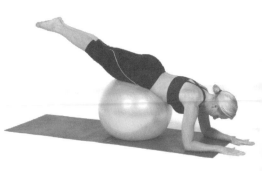

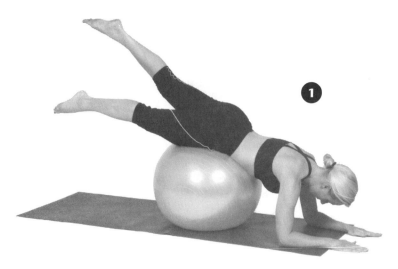

1 As you **EXHALE**, lift your left leg slightly as you lower your right leg slightly. Think about elongating them from your lower back down to your toes.

BEGINNING

Roll the ball farther back so that your thighs are supported by it. This will give you more stability.

variations

2 **INHALE** and switch so that the right leg is higher than the left. Continue to lift and lower your legs on every **INHALE** and **EXHALE**. Two "kicks" equal one rep.

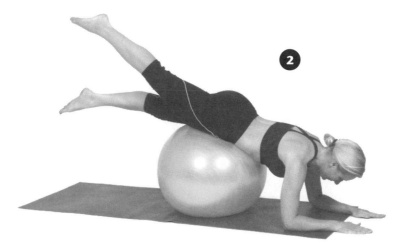

ADVANCED

Extend your arms straight out in front of you.

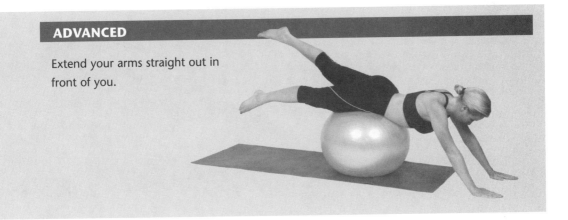

opposition raise

This movement is both a stabilization and movement exercise. Your core works to keep your body in position on the ball and, as your arms and legs move, different muscles of your back and abs are engaged.

STARTING POSITION: Drape your body over the ball, placing your hands flat on the floor. Extend your legs straight out behind you, pointing your toes so that the tops of your feet are on the floor. Your head, neck and shoulders should form one line, and your wrists should be aligned with your shoulders. Gaze at the space between your hands. **INHALE** to begin.

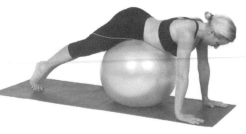

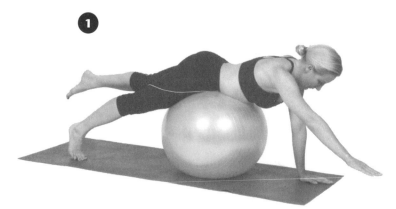

1 As you **EXHALE**, simultaneously raise your right hand and left foot off the floor. The movement is slight: You only need to raise the opposite hand and foot a few inches off the floor. Imagine a person in front of you and behind you, pulling each limb away from your body.

variations

BEGINNING

From the starting position, raise only your right hand off the ground. Return it to the floor and raise your right foot. Continue alternating from right hand then foot to left hand then foot.

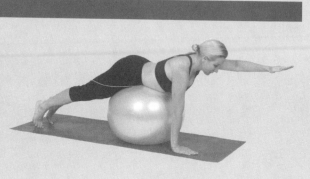

TIPS

- Keep your head aligned with your neck—lifting it or tucking it can stress the tendons in your neck and back.
- Raise your hand and feet no higher than your body. Extending them any higher may stress your back.

2 **INHALE** and lower the hand and foot to the floor. Repeat on the other side.

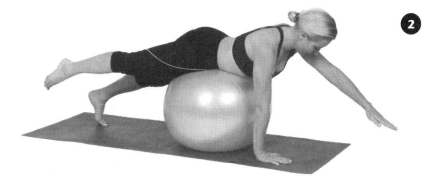

2

ADVANCED

Raise the hand and foot to shoulder and hip height, holding the raise for 5 to 10 full counts.

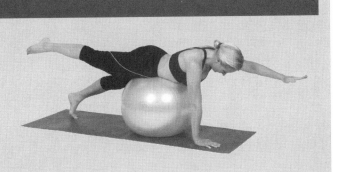

back extension

Your lower back works to raise your upper body in this exercise, while your abs engage to stabilize the ball. The movement is minimal but you'll feel your back working with just a few reps. Maintaining spinal alignment is a must on this exercise, and slow movement will help ensure that.

STARTING POSITION: Kneel behind the ball with your legs hip-width apart. Drape your body over the ball and roll it slightly forward, extending your legs straight out behind you, toes pulled back so that you're balanced on the balls of your feet. Cross your arms high on your chest and bend forward so that your body is curved over the ball.

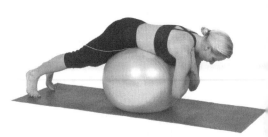

1

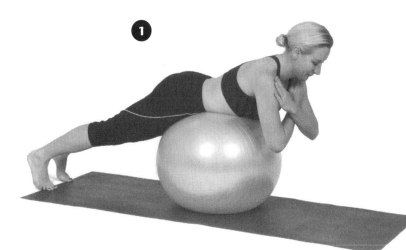

1 INHALE and take two counts to raise your torso slightly until your entire upper body is on the same horizontal plane. Only raise to a point of tension, not strain. Think about a plane taking off—that's the position your upper body should emulate, with your head being the nose of the plane.

variations

BEGINNING

Perform this exercise with your knees bent or feet spread wider apart. This will give you a more stable base.

INTERMEDIATE

Perform this exercise with your legs together and hands holding a dumbbell in front of your chest.

2 **EXHALE** and take two counts to slowly lower your torso to the starting position.

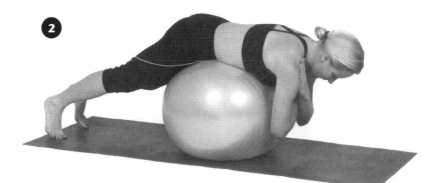

ADVANCED

Hold a dumbbell in both hands and stretch your arms overhead.

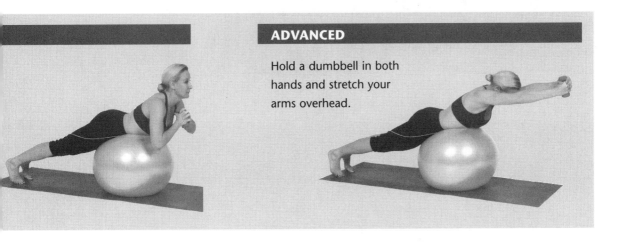

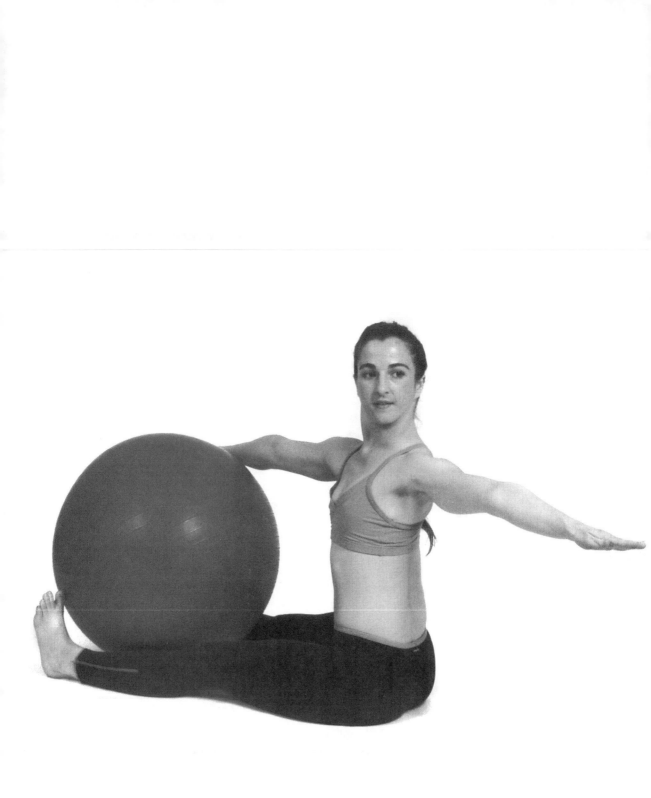

kneeling, standing or sitting on the floor

Whether you're kneeling, standing or sitting, your legs provide a strong base of support for the rest of your body. Although it may seem like your legs do a great deal of the work when you're moving them during some of these exercises, your abs and back are constantly engaged to stabilize you. In fact, that's the way your core muscles are worked in all of these exercises: even if they're not moving, they're stabilizing your body (and keeping you balanced) as other muscle groups move.

side leg lift

This exercise increases your balance and coordination. Your leg muscles work to raise and lower your leg, but your abs stabilize your position and prevent the ball from rolling.

STARTING POSITION: Kneel with the side of one hip against the ball and place the same-side hand on the ball to aid in balance. Extend your outer leg to the side; point your knee forward, rest your arch against the floor, and flex your foot. Place your free hand on your outer thigh or hip for support. Contract your abs and tuck your pelvis slightly to put your spine in a neutral position. Take a moment to get comfortable and stabilize yourself before you move the leg.

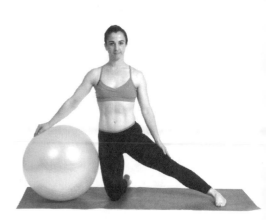

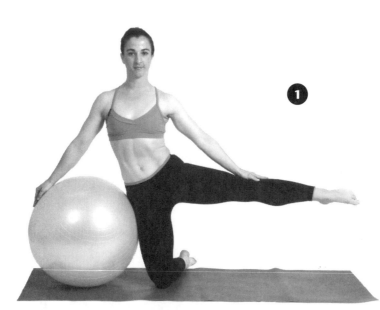

1

1 Keeping your upper body still, **INHALE** and extend your straight leg as you lift it to hip height. Keep your hips square: be careful not to allow the moving leg to pull your hips forward or back.

variations

INTERMEDIATE

Extend your free arm straight out at a diagonal from your shoulder. As you raise your leg, think about extending your arm even farther.

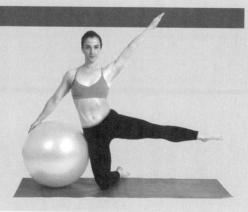

TIPS

• Think about lifting your leg from the hip, not the foot, to help you maintain your alignment.
• Your torso remains still through-out this entire exercise. If you feel your upper body moving, decrease the height of the lift.

2 **EXHALE** as you lower the leg with control to the starting position.

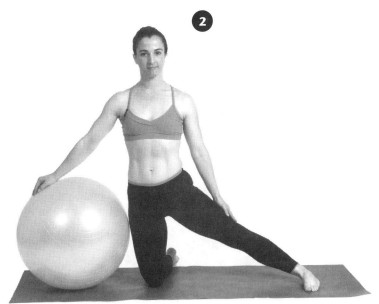

ADVANCED

Straighten both legs out to the side, stacking your feet on top of each other and keeping your knees facing forward. Either place your outer hand on the ball or, for more of a challenge, extend it out as in the intermediate variation. Then proceed to lift the top leg to hip height.

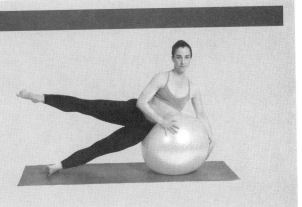

roll-out

Rolling the ball forward in front of you increases the demand on your spine and core muscles to support it. You'll feel the effects of this subtle movement most in your abs.

STARTING POSITION: Kneel behind the ball. Lean slightly forward and place your forearms on top of the ball with your fingers interlaced. Tuck your elbows in close to your sides. Point your toes so that the tops of your feet are resting on the floor and angle your hips slightly forward so that your body forms a diagonal line from your knees to your head. Gaze straight ahead to maintain proper head and spine alignment. **INHALE** to begin.

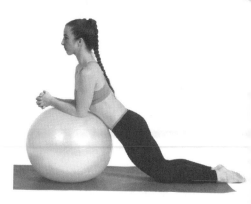

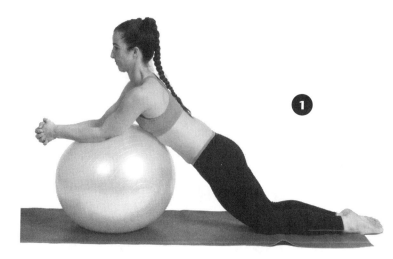

1

1 As you **EXHALE**, slowly roll the ball forward as your elbows push away from your body, contracting your abs to keep your back elongated and not rounded.

variations

INTERMEDIATE

Instead of working from your knees, extend your legs straight out behind you, slightly wider than hip-width apart, and tuck your toes so you're on the balls of your feet. Gaze at your hands. Leaning on your forearms, roll the ball forward and back slightly.

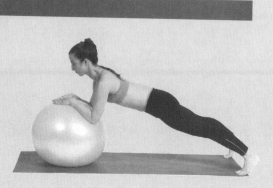

TIPS

- Resist the urge to arch your back as you roll the ball forward.
- If the ball feels like it's rolling out from beneath you, press down on it with your forearms and elbows to help keep it steady.
- Think about keeping your torso completely still as your elbows move away and return to it.

2 As you **INHALE**, pull your elbows in to roll the ball back to the starting position.

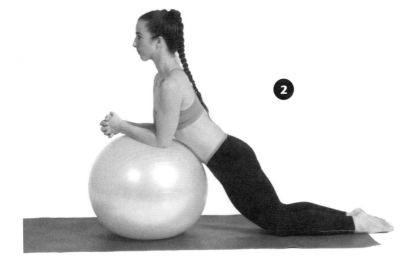

2

ADVANCED

Extend your legs straight out behind you, slightly wider than hip-width apart, as in the intermediate version. Place your hands, not your forearms, on top of the ball. Push down on the ball with your hands as you roll it out and pull it in. Gaze down at the space between your hands.

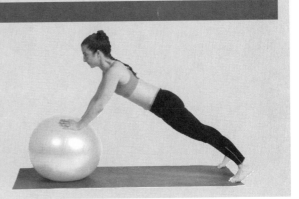

kneeling rotation

You'll work your obliques and stretch your spine as your body twists in this rotation exercise. You can also use this exercise as a stretch for your spine and shoulders: simply hold each rotation for a few breaths instead of twisting continuously from side to side.

STARTING POSITION: Kneel behind the ball. Place your palms on the side of the ball and contract your abs to put your spine in a neutral position. Keeping your spine neutral and your abs contracted, sit back on your heels as you lean slightly forward and the ball rolls away from you. Your head is relaxed between your arms and your hands are resting on the ball. **INHALE** to begin.

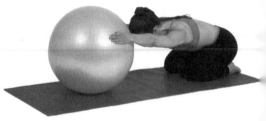

INTERMEDIATE/ADVANCED

As you rotate and open your body to the left, remove your right arm from the ball and reach it under your left arm. Return it to the ball and repeat with the opposite arm.

variations

target: obliques, spine extensors

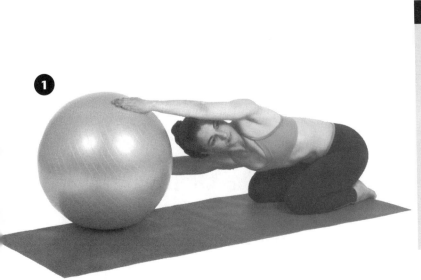

1

1 As you **EXHALE**, rotate your torso and roll the ball to the right. Your body opens up to the left side, but your butt remains on your heels. Keep your head aligned with your neck even in the twisted position so as to not strain your neck.

2 **INHALE** and return to center; repeat to the other side.

2

side crunch

This exercise works the sides of your waist isometrically as you hold your position on the ball, and actively as you lift and lower your torso.

STARTING POSITION: Kneel with your left hip against the ball, left forearm on top of the ball for support. Lean against the ball and roll it slightly so that your hip and waist are resting against it. Extend your right leg straight out to your side with your knee and toes pointing forward. Place your hand, fingers unclasped, behind your head.

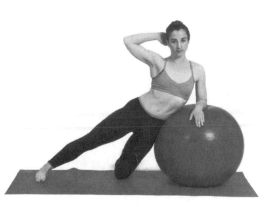

1

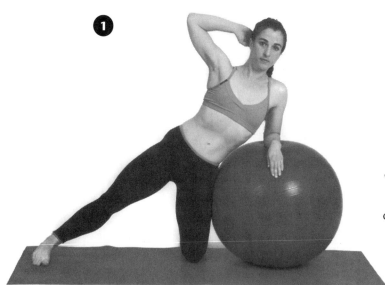

1 **INHALE** and extend your torso to your left so that it drapes over the ball.

variations

BEGINNING

Sitting with your left hip next to the ball, sweep your legs to the right so that your knees are in front of you. Place your left forearm on top of the ball and lean slightly against the ball.

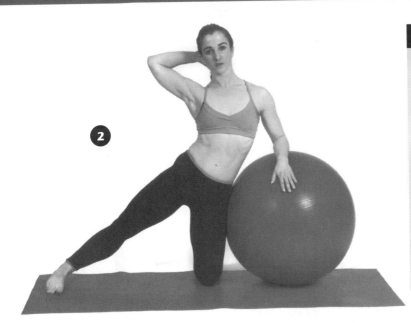

2 EXHALE and lift your torso toward the right, bringing the right side of your ribcage toward your right hip. Keep your lower body still throughout the movement.

TIPS

- Think about shortening the distance between your ribs and hips as you crunch up to your side. Lift up through your opposite side to extend down to the other.
- Your head, chest and hips face forward. Your body should not fall forward or back as you move.
- Be careful not to pull on your head with your hands, as this can strain your neck.

3 Return to the Step 1 position and repeat all reps before switching sides.

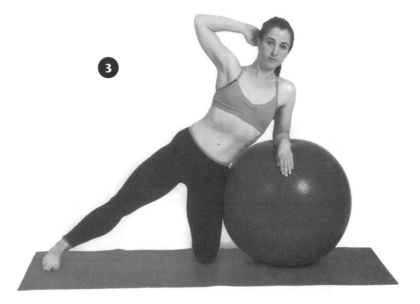

around the world

By taking your back and abs through a circular range of motion, you'll work all of the two body parts' muscles at once. Your hamstrings will also get a good stretch, which can help alleviate lower back pain and stiffness.

STARTING POSITION: Stand with your legs spread fairly wide apart, holding the ball overhead. There should be a small space between the ball and your head. Contract your abs so your spine is in a neutral position. Your head, neck and shoulders are aligned. **INHALE** deeply to begin, as you'll need to exhale for the entire rotation.

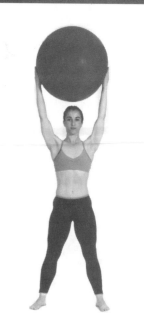

1

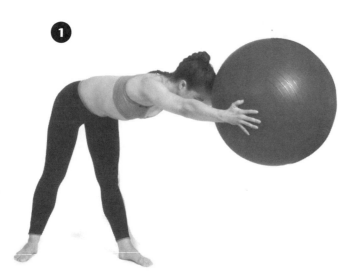

1 As you **EXHALE**, simultaneously lift your torso as you turn it toward your left side, keeping your hips facing forward. Hinging at your hips, bend forward to bring your chest toward your left thigh.

variations

BEGINNING

Begin holding the ball in front of you at chest height. Rotate and return to this position.

2

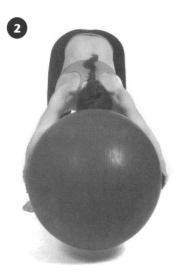

2 Staying bent with your back elongated, rotate counter-clockwise, bringing your torso between your legs and then toward your right thigh.

3 Continue rotating until you're standing upright in the start position with the ball overhead. Repeat all reps before rotating toward the opposite side.

3

ADVANCED

Perform the exercise while holding a 2- to 3-pound dumbbell in each hand, pressing your forearms against the ball to hold it.

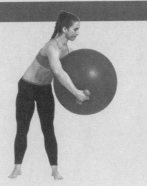

straight-leg deadlift

Since weak or tight hamstrings can contribute to back pain, it's helpful to include exercises that strengthen and stretch them in your core-training routine.

STARTING POSITION: Stand with your legs hip-width apart and straight, but not locked. Your head, shoulders and hips are aligned. Wrap both arms around the ball and squeeze your arms, as if you were hugging the ball. (The ball will be touching your chest.) Contract your abs to elongate your torso. **INHALE** to begin.

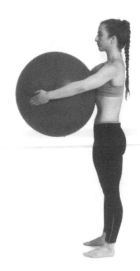

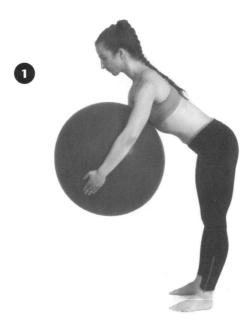

1 Slightly push your hips back. As you **EXHALE**, bend forward at your waist so that the ball lowers toward the floor. Your back should remain straight and elongated.

variations

BEGINNING

If you lack flexibility in your hamstrings, perform this exercise with a slight bend in your knees and arms.

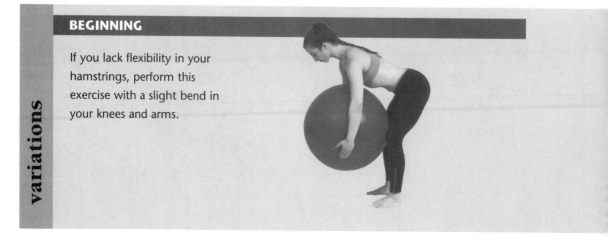

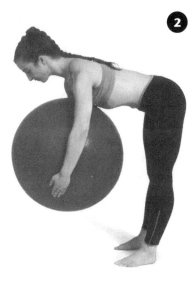

2 Lower only to the point where you feel a stretch behind your legs (any further is unsafe and can cause you to strain your back or hamstrings). If you're more flexible, lower until your upper body is parallel to the floor.

TIPS

- Pushing your hips back before bending will help ensure you're hinging your body at your hips, not your torso.
- Keep your shoulders pulled back throughout the lowering and lifting phases.
- Imagine you're hugging a tree as you're holding the ball.

3 As you **INHALE**, pull through your hamstrings and lower back to raise your upper body to the starting position. Immediately move into your next rep.

ADVANCED

Hold a 2- to 3-pound dumbbell in each hand, palms facing forward, and squeeze the ball between your forearms.

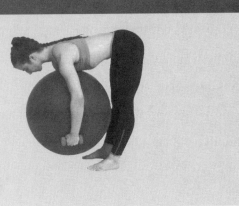

seated straddle twist

Rotating increases your spine's mobility and flexibility. Positioning your legs in a straddle stretches your hamstrings, which can help relieve lower back pain and stiffness.

STARTING POSITION: Sit on the floor and extend your legs out in front of you. Place the ball between your calves and tighten your leg muscles to hold the ball in place. Flex your feet and point your toes and knees toward the ceiling. Extend your arms straight out to your sides into a T with your palms face down. **INHALE** and elongate your spine to begin.

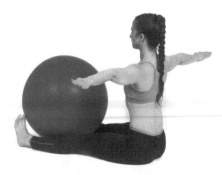

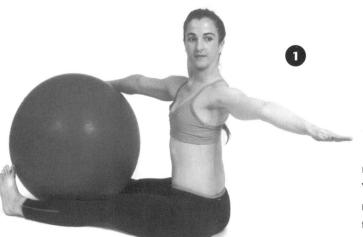

1

1 As you **EXHALE**, rotate your torso to the left until your right hand touches the ball. Your hips shouldn't lift as you rotate—concentrate on keeping them pressed against the floor.

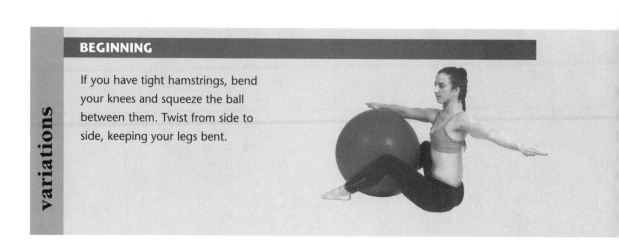

variations

BEGINNING

If you have tight hamstrings, bend your knees and squeeze the ball between them. Twist from side to side, keeping your legs bent.

2 **INHALE** to return to the starting position; repeat to the other side.

2

ADVANCED

Position the ball closer to your toes. As you rotate, lean slightly forward. This will increase the rotation of your spine.

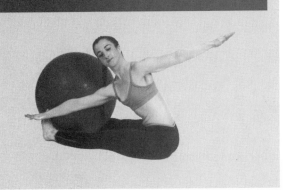

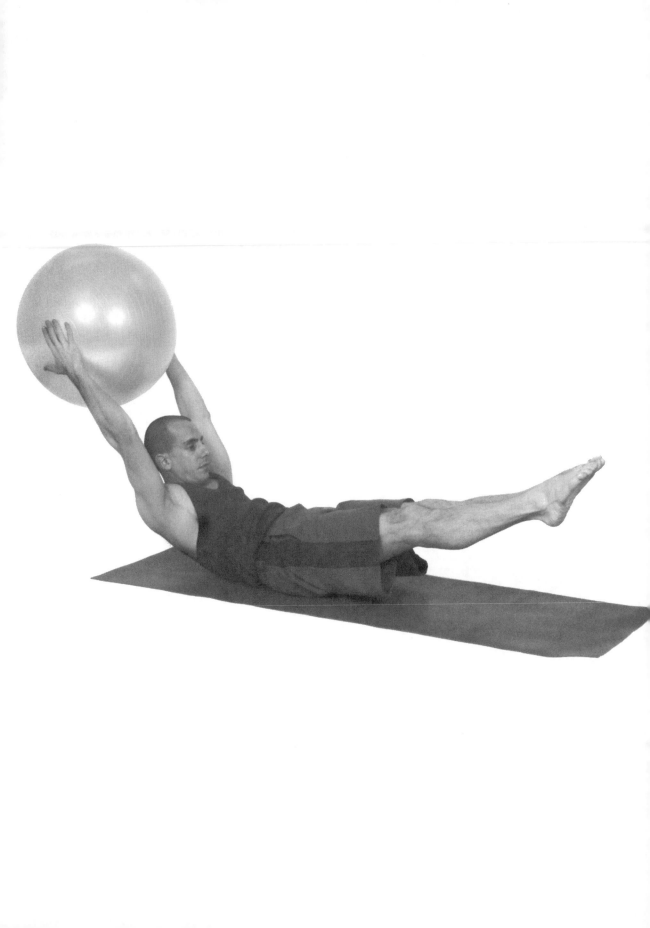

lying on the floor, ball at head

Holding the ball overhead and lifting your shoulder blades off the floor immediately engages your abs. When you simultaneously lift your upper and lower body—as you will in many of the exercises in this section— you force the opposing muscle groups of your abs and back to work together. This not only strengthens your core, it also improves your posture.

scissors

If you have a neck injury, do not attempt this movement.

STARTING POSITION: Hold the ball with both hands and lie on your back. Curl both knees into your chest and rest the ball on your shins.

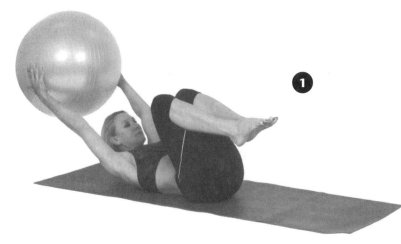

1 **INHALE** and raise your head, neck and shoulders off the floor, extending your arms and the ball straight above your head. Keep your head, neck and shoulders raised throughout the exercise, and keep your abs flat. You should not see your abdomen push out as you curl forward. Your arms are straight, but your elbows are not locked.

variations

BEGINNING

When you split your legs, bend one leg into your chest and touch the ball to its shin. Repeat with the opposite leg, always keeping one leg bent.

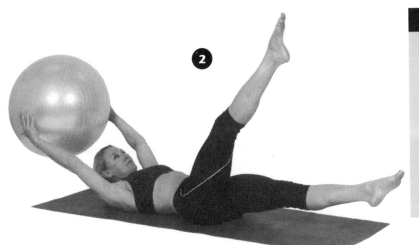

2 As you **EXHALE**, simultaneously straighten and split your legs so that your right leg is raised and your left leg is lowered. **INHALE**.

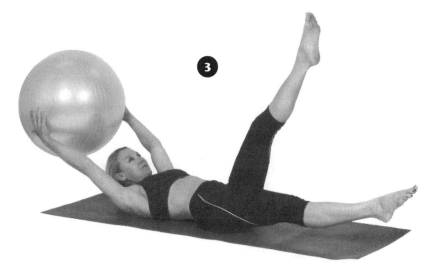

3 As you **EXHALE**, switch leg position so that the left leg is raised and the right leg drops toward the floor. Continue alternating the top leg with each breath.

ADVANCED

Eliminate the scissors movement and instead do a V-up. As you lift your head and shoulder blades off the floor, simultaneously straighten and raise your legs while bringing your arms forward until the ball touches your shins. Lower your upper and lower body until they're one inch off the floor.

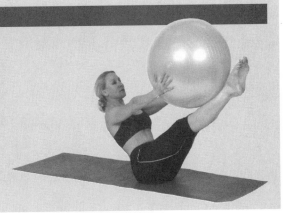

roll-up

In addition to strengthening the abs, this move stretches the leg muscles. This exercise is best performed in a flowing motion, with no rest between reps.

STARTING POSITION: Lie on your back with your legs hip-width apart and stretched out along the floor. Your feet should be pointed and your legs should feel elongated throughout the exercise. Hold the ball overhead with both arms extended behind you. Draw your shoulder blades down your back. **INHALE** to begin.

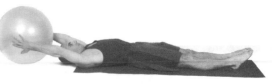

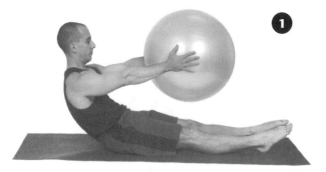

1 As you **EXHALE**, pull your upper body off the floor and lift the ball up and forward until your arms are straight out in front of your chest. Don't allow your shoulders to hunch forward as you roll up.

BEGINNING

Perform the roll-up with your knees bent, feet flat on the ground.

variations

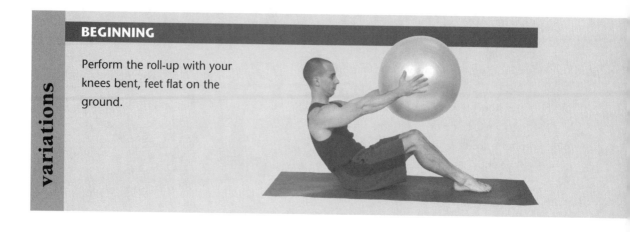

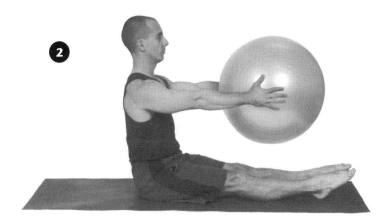

2

2 Continue raising your body until you're seated upright, arms extended straight out in front of your chest. Your head, neck, shoulders and hips are aligned.

3 Immediately begin slowly rolling back to the starting position, allowing one vertebra at a time to touch the floor. When the ball touches the floor behind you, immediately move into the next roll-up.

TIPS

- Perform this exercise at the end of your workout when you're most flexible.
- If your hamstrings or back feel tight, bend your knees and place your feet flat on the floor.
- Use your breathing to guide you from the reclined position to the upright one and back again.
- If you find yourself hunching, perform a few reps without the ball to get comfortable with the positioning.

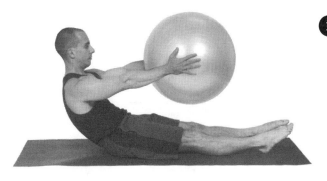

3

ADVANCED

When you reach the upright seated position, continue bending forward, pushing the ball toward your feet. Then slowly roll back to the starting position.

straight-body crunch

Keeping your legs extended straight out in front of you places most of the workload on your upper abs.

STARTING POSITION: Lie on your back with your legs extended along the floor. Hold the ball with both hands and extend your arms above your head so that your elbows frame your ears. Imagine extending your body through your toes and the tips of your fingers. Maintain this elongated position throughout the exercise. Contract your abs and press your lower back into the floor. **INHALE** to begin.

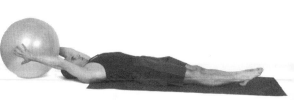

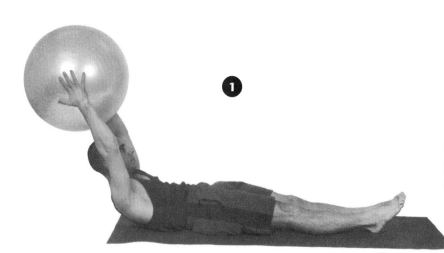

1 As you **EXHALE**, lift your head and shoulder blades off the floor. Keep the ball directly overhead or slightly behind it and your head and neck aligned. Don't allow your belly to protrude out as you lift your shoulder blades, as this can strain your lower back. Continue pressing your lower back into the floor to prevent this.

variations

BEGINNING

Place your feet on the floor, slightly wider than hip-width apart, and bend your knees. Hold the ball with both hands and extend your arms above your head so that your elbows are at your ears. Keeping your arms straight, raise and lower your head and shoulder blades.

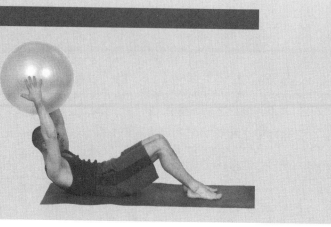

TIPS

• Holding the ball overhead makes it more difficult to maintain your head, neck and shoulder alignment. If you feel yourself pulling forward with your arms, try a few reps without the ball.

• Don't pull on your neck as you lift. Imagine that your head, neck, shoulders and the ball are fused together. Lift and lower them as one unit, maintaining their alignment.

2 **INHALE** as you lower to the starting position.

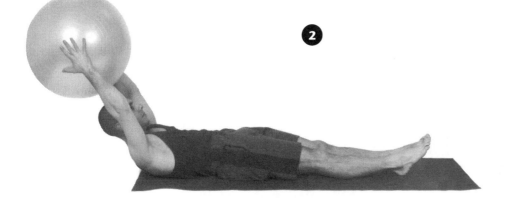

❷

ADVANCED

Raise your straight legs 45 degrees off the floor and keep them in that position as you lift and lower your shoulder blades off the floor.

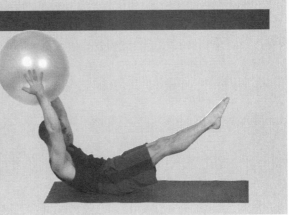

straight-body oblique crunch

The subtle side-to-side raise activates the deepest parts of your obliques, as well as the difficult-to-reach transverse abdominis.

STARTING POSITION: Lie on your back with your legs extended along the floor. Hold the ball with both hands and extend your arms above your head, elbows by your ears. Contract your abs and press your lower back into the floor. **INHALE** to begin.

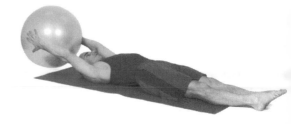

1 As you **EXHALE**, lift both shoulder blades off the floor and twist toward the right side of the room. Keep the ball directly overhead or slightly behind it and your head and neck aligned. Your hips stay perfectly still and pressed into the floor as you lift. The movement comes only from your upper body.

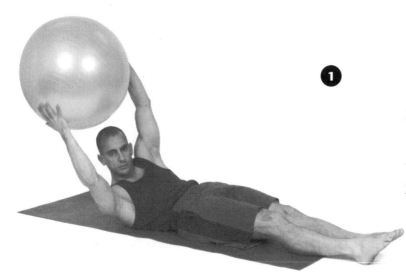

variations

BEGINNING

Lie on your back and bend your knees, placing your feet flat on the floor. Maintain this position as you lift and lower your shoulder blades.

TIPS

- Although you're raising your body toward one side, both shoulder blades should be lifted off the floor—one will just be lifted slightly higher as you rotate.
- The movement consists of a fluid lift and rotation. Lift before you rotate to ensure you activate the abs properly.

2 **INHALE** and return to the starting position, then **EXHALE** and lift both shoulder blades off the floor, twisting toward the left side of the room.

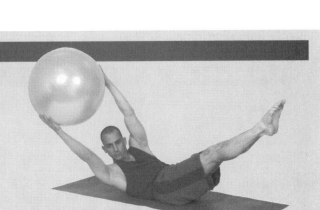

2

ADVANCED

Raise your straight legs about 45 degrees off the floor. Keep them in this position as you lift your shoulder blades toward the right and then the left.

superman

Lifting your arms and feet from a completely flat position is very difficult, but it simultaneously works every muscle along your spine as well as your rectus abdominis. In the lifted position, your body will be in the flying position of the superhero for which this exercise is named.

STARTING POSITION: Lie face down on the floor with the ball just above your head. Grasp the ball with both hands. Keeping your legs together, straighten them and point your toes. Press the tops of your feet against the floor. **INHALE** to begin.

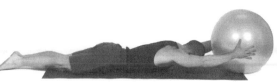

1 As you **EXHALE**, contract your abs to raise your arms to shoulder height, which will raise the uppermost part of your torso off the floor. Simultaneously contract your butt to lift your lower legs just past hip height. Hold for one to two counts.

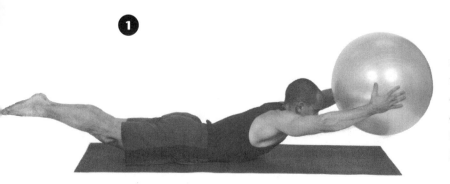

variations

BEGINNING

Keep your legs pressed against the floor and only lift your arms, head and shoulders off the floor.

TIPS

- Your lower back shouldn't arch past its point of normal curvature. Contracting your abs as you lift will help protect your lower back.
- Think about opening your chest as your arms lift off the floor to alleviate some of the pressure on your lower back.
- Keep your shoulder blades pulled down and relaxed as you lift and lower.

2 **INHALE** and lower your body to the floor.

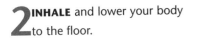

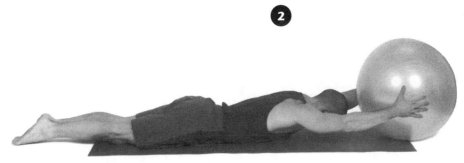

ADVANCED

Place 2- to 3-pound ankle weights around your ankles. The added resistance will make the exercise harder.

leg crosses

Your lower abs must work to pulsate your legs back and forth. The repetitive motion of the leg crossing will also raise your heart rate, which means you'll also get an aerobic challenge when doing this exercise.

STARTING POSITION: Lie on your back with your legs extended along the floor. Hold the ball with both hands and extend your arms overhead. Contract your abs to press your lower back into the floor. Lift your head, neck and shoulders off the floor and lift your legs so that they're about 45 degrees off the floor. **INHALE** to begin.

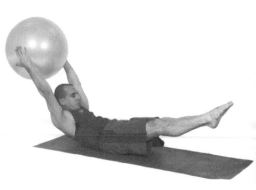

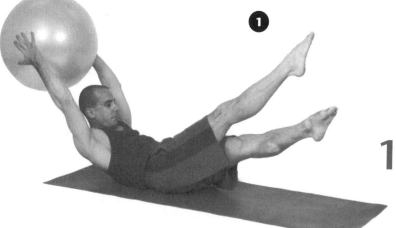

1

1 **EXHALE** and cross your right leg over your left.

variations

BEGINNING

Bend your legs so that your shins are parallel to the ground. Cross your legs over each other at the knee, maintaining the bend for the entire exercise.

2 Open your legs and cross your left over your right. Continue, criss-crossing legs and alternating the top leg. Breathe at a comfortable rate—don't hold your breath!

TIPS

- Draw your shoulder blades down and keep your elbows aligned with your ears to prevent stress on your back.
- Periodically look down at your belly and make sure it's not protruding. Continually contract your abs and press your lower back into the floor to prevent this.
- If you feel any pain in your neck, perform this exercise without the ball—keep your head, neck and shoulders down against the floor, arms straight down alongside your body.

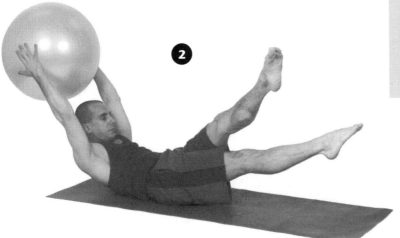

2

ADVANCED

Perform the exercise with your legs hovering about two inches above the floor. The closer your legs are to the ground, the harder the exercise is.

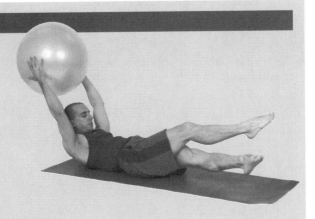

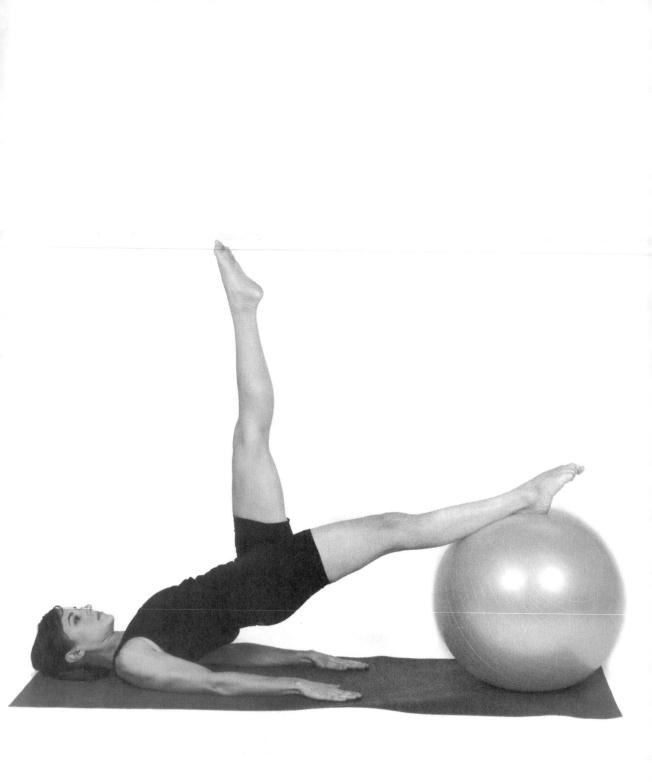

lying on the floor, ball at feet

Lying on the floor eliminates the automatic activation of your core muscles that occurs in many other positions, but it doesn't make these exercises easier than those in other sections. These movements all require the active participation of the muscles of your abs and back to move your legs, hips or upper body. While the range of motion from this position may seem small, the workload goes deep.

crunch with feet on ball

Elevating your feet on the ball in this version of the crunch puts greater stress on the upper part of your abs.

STARTING POSITION: Lie on your back with your knees bent 90 degrees and draped over the ball so your thighs are perpendicular to the floor. (To keep the ball stationary, you may position it against a wall.) Press your heels into the ball to keep it in place. Place your hands, fingers unclasped, behind your head. Contract your abs to put your spine in a neutral position. **INHALE** to begin.

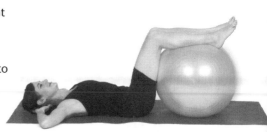

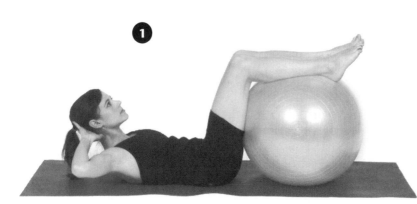

1 As you **EXHALE**, slowly raise your shoulder blades off the floor without pulling on your head or neck. Think about shortening the space between your hips and chest while simultaneously keeping your head aligned with your neck. Hold the contraction at the top of the movement.

INTERMEDIATE

Perform the same movement with your arms stretched overhead, one hand holding the wrist of the opposite hand.

variations

TIPS

- It is especially difficult to maintain the natural curvature of your back as you lower to the starting position, so take a moment to realign your body if necessary.
- Straightening your legs and resting your calves on the ball increases the stability challenge.

2 **INHALE** as you slowly lower your shoulder blades to the floor, then immediately move into the next rep. Your back should maintain its natural curve, but not arch.

2

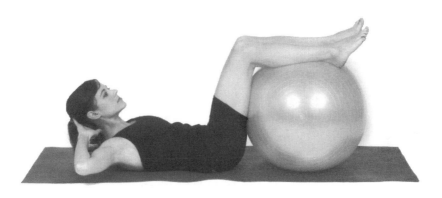

ADVANCED

Hold a dumbbell at your chest while performing the exercise. The added resistance increases the intensity for your abs.

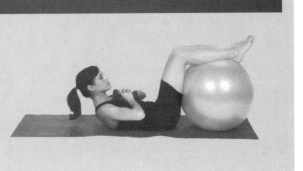

oblique crunch with feet on ball

The rising phase of the exercise consists of two parts—lifting and twisting—but they should be performed in one fluid motion.

STARTING POSITION: Lie on your back with your legs resting on top of the ball, knees bent 90 degrees so that your thighs are perpendicular to the floor. (To keep the ball stationary, you may position it against a wall.) Press your heels into the ball to keep it in place. Place your hands, fingers unclasped, behind your head. Contract your abs to put your spine in a neutral position. **INHALE** to begin.

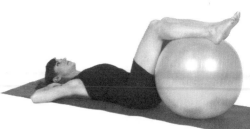

1

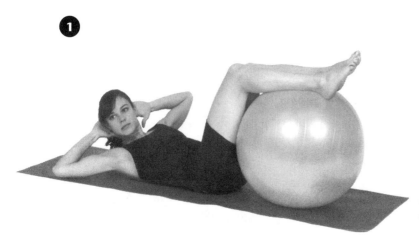

1 As you **EXHALE**, raise your shoulder blades off the floor, being careful not to pull on your neck, and twist your left shoulder toward your right knee.

variations

INTERMEDIATE

As you lift one shoulder off the floor, lift the opposite bent leg toward it. The knee and elbow shouldn't meet—you are lifting your shoulder, not your elbow, toward your knee.

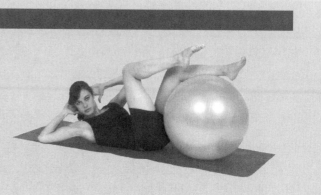

TIPS

- Think about raising your shoulder, not your elbow, to meet the opposite knee to help prevent you from pulling on your neck as you twist.
- When you twist, feel the oblique of the side you're twisting toward contract. If you're not sure if you're contracting the muscle, put your hand on it as you perform a rep. You should feel it tightening.

2 **INHALE** as you untwist and lower to the starting position. Repeat to the other side.

2

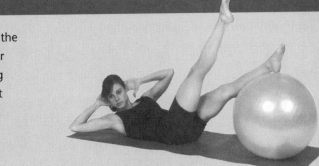

ADVANCED

Straighten your legs and roll the ball forward so that only your calves rest on it. As you bring one shoulder off the floor, lift your opposite leg, keeping it straight.

reverse crunch

Curling your hips toward your chest forces the lower abs to engage.

STARTING POSITION: Lie on your back with your legs bent over the ball. Place your arms along your sides, palms facing down. Press your lower abs into the floor to stabilize your back. Press your heels into the ball and hold it between your feet and buttocks. **INHALE** to begin.

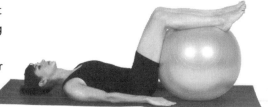

1 While squeezing the ball, **EXHALE** as you slowly raise your knees toward your chest, lifting your hips slightly off the floor.

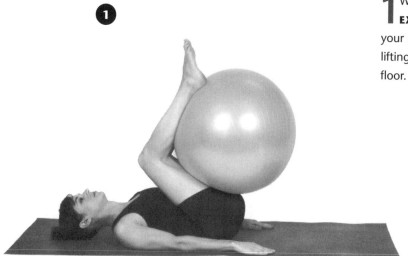

variations

BEGINNING

Begin with your knees bent and hold the ball between them by squeezing your thighs.

TIPS

- Concentrate on keeping your lower back pressed against the floor. This is especially challenging as you return your legs to the starting position.
- Use your abs, not the momentum of the movement, to lift and lower your hips. Swinging your knees up and down takes the work away from the target muscles and also strains your back.

2 Slowly lower your hips and the ball to the starting position. Don't allow your muscles to relax as you lower your legs. Immediately curl your hips into the next rep.

2

ADVANCED

Begin with your hands unclasped behind your head. Lift your shoulder blades off the floor as your knees come toward your chest. Lower your shoulder blades to the floor as you lower your feet to the floor.

reverse crunch twist

This exercise targets the lower-most part of your abs and your obliques. Your spine extensors work to twist your hips.

STARTING POSITION: Lie on your back with your legs bent over the ball. Place your arms along your sides, palms facing down. Press your lower abs into the floor to stabilize your back. Press your heels into the ball and hold it between your feet and buttocks. **INHALE** to begin.

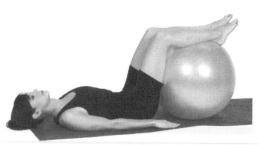

1 While squeezing the ball with your heels, **EXHALE** and pull your knees up toward your chest as you simultaneously lift and rotate your hips to one side. The ball will lift slightly off the floor.

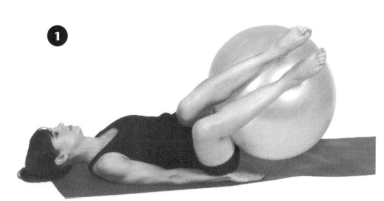

BEGINNING

Instead of pulling your knees in toward your chest, rotate them to one side as your opposite hip raises slightly off the floor. The ball will roll slightly as your knees move. Return to center and rotate your knees to the other side.

variations

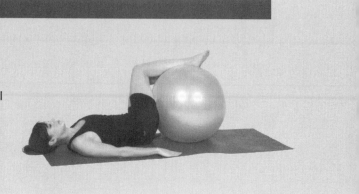

TIPS

- If your lower back arches when you're lowering your legs, you're relaxing your abs. Concentrate on pressing your back against the floor to keep your abs tight.
- Try not to use momentum to lift and lower your legs. Moving slowly through both phases of the movement will ensure the workload stays on your core instead of your legs.

2 **INHALE** and lower your legs to the starting position. Repeat to the other side.

2

ADVANCED

Place your hands, fingers unclasped, behind your head. As you twist your hips to the left, curl your left shoulder toward your right knee. This intensifies the abdominal contraction.

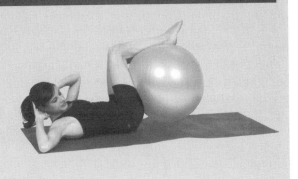

bridge

The traditional yoga bridge pose is performed with both legs bent, feet flat on the ground. Placing your legs atop the ball better engages your abs as it forces them to contract to stabilize your spine.

STARTING POSITION: Lie on your back and, with legs extended, rest your calves on top of the ball. Your arms are along your sides and your palms are facing down. **INHALE** to begin.

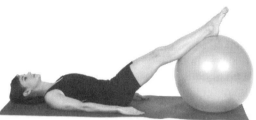

1 As you **EXHALE**, tilt your pelvis and then raise your hips off the floor until they're diagonally aligned with your shoulders.

1

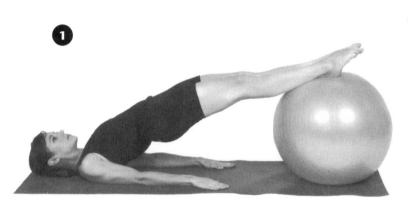

variations

INTERMEDIATE

As you raise your hips off the floor, bend one leg so that it comes off the ball. Return it to the starting position and lift the opposite leg with the next rep.

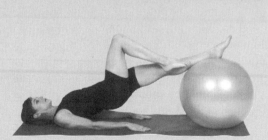

TIPS

- If it's difficult to stabilize yourself, move the ball closer to your torso. You can also bend your legs over the ball.
- Your back shouldn't arch in the elevated position. Think about thrusting your hips forward to help keep your hips in line with your body.
- Don't allow your shoulders to hunch forward. Before you begin, think about rolling your shoulder blades down your upper back.
- The bridge also works the hamstrings. After doing a few reps, you may want to do a seated hamstring stretch to relax the muscles.

2 **INHALE** as you slowly lower your body—back and then hips—to the starting position.

2

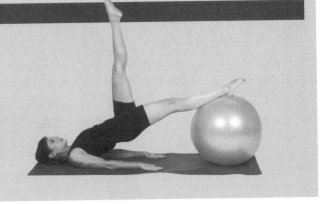

ADVANCED

As you raise your hips off the floor, extend one leg straight up toward the ceiling. Keep it extended as you complete all reps and extend the opposite leg for your next set.

lying leg rotation

Your spine extensors work to push and pull your body when rotating, but you'll feel this exercise most in your obliques.

STARTING POSITION: Lie on the floor with your legs bent and the ball between your knees. Extend your arms straight out to your sides into a T. Raise your bent legs, hugging the ball between them. Your head, neck and shoulders are relaxed. Contract your abs to bring your spine into a neutral position and press your lower back into the floor.

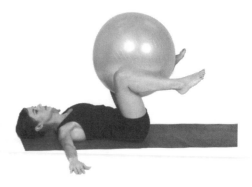

1

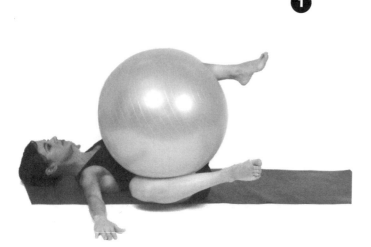

1 Keeping both shoulder blades pressed into the floor, **INHALE** as you lower your knees toward one side of your body, letting your hips roll slightly as well.

variations

BEGINNING

Start out by doing this exercise without the ball. When you're comfortable, add the ball.

2 **EXHALE** as you use your obliques to pull your knees back to center. Repeat to the other side.

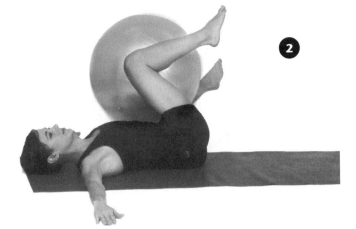

ADVANCED

Begin with your legs straight and the ball between your calves, toes pointing toward the ceiling. Rotate your hips to one side, allowing your legs to drop toward the floor.

legs overhead

Since there's no pause between the lifting and lowering phases of the movement, you maintain a constant ab contraction, which means you work the muscle group equally hard throughout all parts of the exercise.

STARTING POSITION: Lie on the floor with your legs straight, squeezing the ball between your calves. Extend your arms along your sides and relax your head and neck. Contract your abs to press your lower back into the floor.

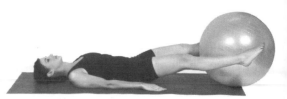

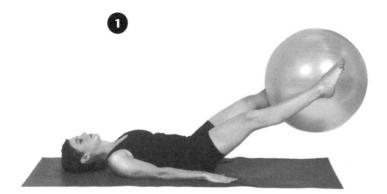

1

1 **INHALE** and use your abs to raise your legs. Press your palms into the floor to help stabilize your position.

variations

INTERMEDIATE/ADVANCED

Keep your legs slightly bent (like frog legs) throughout the movement. When your legs are overhead, your knees will be near your head.

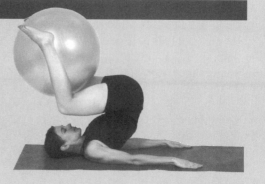

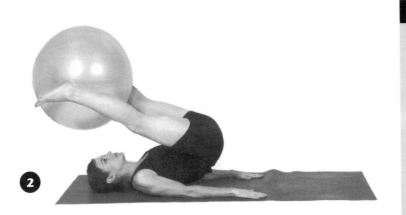

2 When your feet and the ball reach the point where they're 90 degrees from the floor, lift your hips slightly to continue pushing them until they're over your head.

3 **EXHALE** as you lower your body—touching one vertebra at a time to the floor—until your hips reach the floor and your legs are straight up in the air (forming right angles to the floor). Then immediately begin the next rep.

TIPS

- Don't roll onto your neck. Only roll the ball back to the point where your middle back is off the floor; your shoulder blades and upper back are always in contact with the floor.
- As your legs move overhead, think about reaching the ball to the wall behind you.
- If you're lowering your legs beyond the point where they're perpendicular to the floor, stop at the point where your lower back starts to arch. Going any farther will strain your lower back.

ADVANCED

Continue lowering your legs until they reach the starting position or a level just above the floor. Then move into the next rep.

straight-leg hip roll

The subtle movement of rotating your lower body while stabilizing your upper body really targets the lower sides of your waist.

STARTING POSITION: Lie on your back and place your calves on top of the ball. Point your toes. Your upper body is pressed against the floor and your arms are extended along your sides, palms facing down. Contract your abs and **INHALE** to begin.

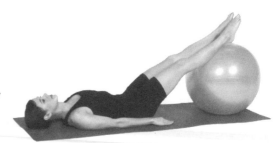

1 EXHALE as you rotate your hips to the right, keeping your legs straight and upper body still.

①

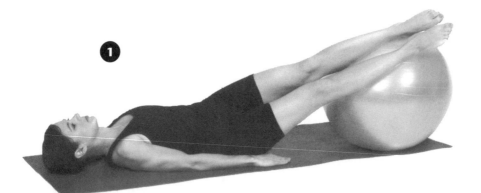

variations

BEGINNING

Perform the hip roll without the ball. Lie on your back with your legs extended straight along the floor, toes pointed and lower back pressed into the floor. Rotate your hips from side to side, keeping both shoulder blades pressed into the floor.

2 **INHALE** and return to center, then repeat to the other side.

Return to the starting position.

2

ADVANCED

Place your hands behind your head, fingers unclasped. As you rotate your hips, raise your head and shoulder blades off the floor. Keep them raised for the entire set.

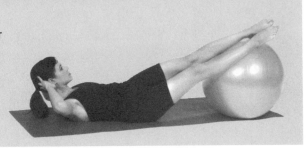

lying straight-leg lifts

You'll be using your lower abs, not your hips and thighs, to raise and lower your legs. Adding the upper body lift makes these leg lifts an upper ab exercise as well.

STARTING POSITION: Lie on your back and place your calves on top of the ball. Point your toes. Your upper body is pressed against the floor, arms straight down at your sides. **INHALE** and bring your arms overhead to begin.

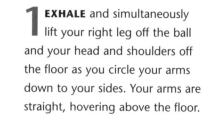

1 **EXHALE** and simultaneously lift your right leg off the ball and your head and shoulders off the floor as you circle your arms down to your sides. Your arms are straight, hovering above the floor.

BEGINNING

Keep your head and shoulders pressed into the floor and only move your arms with your leg.

variations

TIPS

- If your neck feels strained, perform the beginner variation.
- Keep your focus on your belly to prevent your head from falling back or reaching forward.
- Think about reaching out with your fingers as you bring your arms overhead and circle them around to the sides of your body.

2 INHALE and place your leg back on the ball as you return your torso and arms to the starting position. Repeat on the other side.

2

INTERMEDIATE/ADVANCED

To increase the challenge, move the ball farther away from your legs so that only your ankles are resting on it.

double-leg stretch

Don't be afraid to try the advanced variation of this exercise. It requires a bit more coordination, but you'll work up to it quite quickly.

STARTING POSITION: Lie on your back with your knees bent and your feet pressing into the ball. Contract your abs, pressing your lower back into the floor. Extend your arms alongside your body so that your palms are facing in. **INHALE** and lift your head and shoulder blades off the floor.

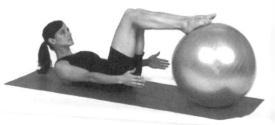

1 As you **EXHALE**, slowly straighten your legs to roll the ball away from you as you raise your arms overhead so that your elbows frame your ears. Don't arch your lower back. This is especially easy to do as you extend your legs, so reassess your form as you stretch your legs.

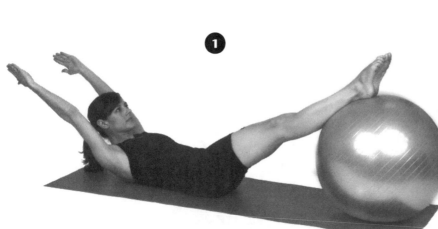

1

variations

BEGINNING

Keep your head and shoulder blades flat on the floor instead of elevating them. This will help you get comfortable with the action of rolling the ball.

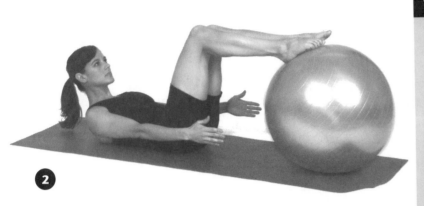

2

2 Keeping your head and shoulder blades lifted, **INHALE** and bend your knees to roll the ball back toward you, circling your arms back to the sides of your hips. Keep your head and shoulder blades elevated for all reps.

TIPS

- Keeping your head and shoulder blades lifted forces your abs to remain contracted.
- Think about moving your arms in a semicircular motion from your head to your hips. Your palms begin facing in, turn out to circle around your body and end facing in near your hips.
- Think about stretching your legs out to the opposite wall and pulling your knees into your chest. Overemphasizing the movement can help you with form and focus.

ADVANCED

As your knees bend and the ball rolls toward you, take one foot off the ball and curl that knee in toward your chest. As you straighten your legs, return the foot to the ball and on the next rep lift the opposite leg.

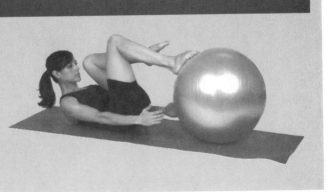

straight-leg bicycles

Bicycles are one of the most effective abs exercises. They also challenge you aerobically, as they're done at a quick, heart-rate-elevating pace.

STARTING POSITION: Lie on your back with the ball between your lower legs. Straighten your legs and point your toes to elongate the muscles. Raise your legs to a point just below 90 degrees to the floor. Place both hands, fingers unclasped, behind your head. Contract your abs, pressing your lower back into the floor, and lift your head, neck and shoulder blades off the floor. **INHALE** to begin.

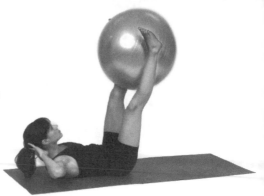

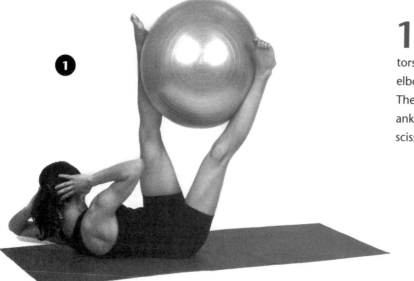

1 As you **EXHALE**, simultaneously twist your torso and hips to reach one elbow toward the opposite knee. The ball rotates between your ankles and your legs twist in a scissor motion.

variations

BEGINNING

Perform the exercise with your legs bent and the ball squeezed between them.

2 **INHALE** and twist your upper and lower body to the opposite side, reaching elbow toward opposite knee. Continue twisting back and forth on every **INHALE** and **EXHALE**, not stopping at the center. One twist to each side equals one rep.

TIPS

- Imagine bringing your shoulder, not your elbow, in to meet the opposite knee. This will help ensure that you are twisting your entire torso, not merely your neck or arms.
- Only lower your shoulder blades to the floor between sets.
- Imagine a large weight pressing your body down from your chest to your abdomen. This area remains pressed into the floor as the areas above and below it twist.
- Your elbow are wide out, like butterfly wings. Pulling them in can put excess strain on your neck and upper back.

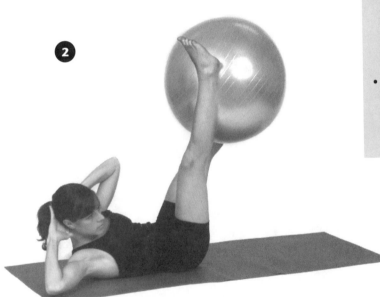

ADVANCED

As you twist, straighten the arm of the side of your torso that's lifting and reach your fingertips (instead of your elbow) toward the opposite ankle (instead of knee).

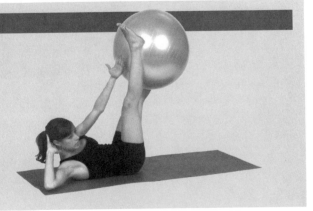

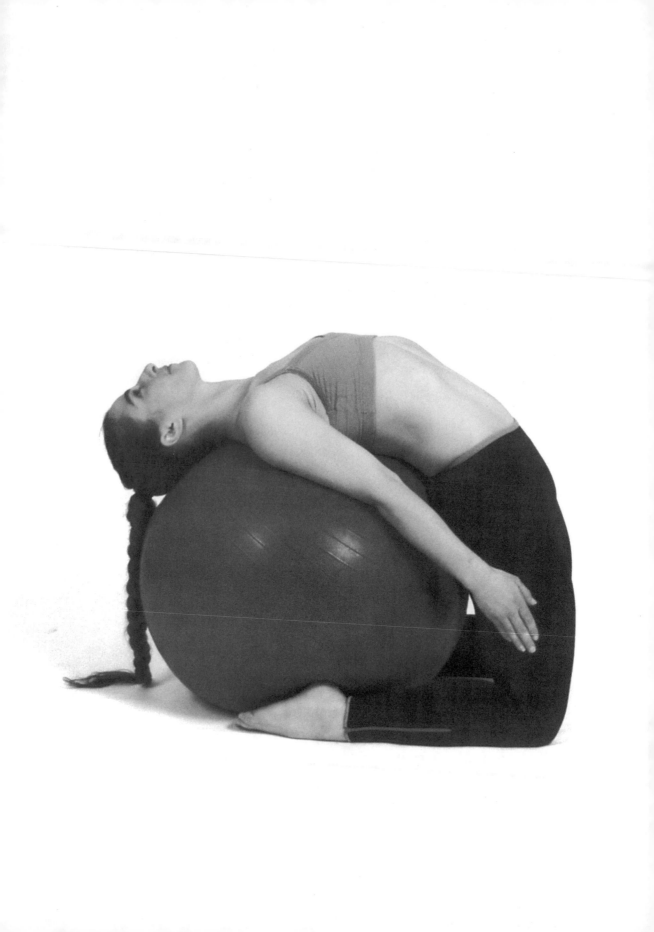

stretches on the ball

Stretching is an important, but often neglected, part of a well-rounded fitness program. When done correctly, it can prevent muscle strain and injury, and improve your flexibility and range of motion. It's especially important when it comes to core training since you're dealing with your back. (Injure or strain your back and you're basically immobile.) As you age, this becomes even more critical. Muscles, like skin, lose elasticity over time and stretching can help keep them more pliable and, thus, you more mobile.

camel pose on the ball

This yoga pose stretches all the muscles on the front of your body, including your abs, and is a strength challenge for your back. If you have lower back or neck pain, do not do this stretch.

STARTING POSITION: Kneel in front of the ball with your thighs perpendicular to the floor and your legs opened slightly wider than hip width (the wider apart your legs are, the easier it is to perform this stretch). Position the ball so that it's between your legs and your butt is pressed against it. Extend your arms along your sides, palms touching the sides of your thighs.

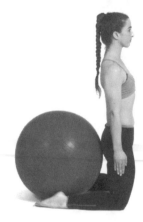

1

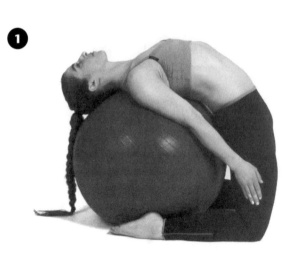

1 Slowly bend back from your hips, allowing your back to curve around the ball. Your arms stay along your sides for support. Relax your head and neck, allowing your head to arch back against the ball. Focus on pushing your pelvis up and forward to prevent your ribcage from jutting out. Hold the stretched position, breathing steadily.

TO COME OUT: Place your hands on the fronts of your hips and lift your head and torso off the ball by pushing your hips forward. Lead with your chest, not your head, as you come up.

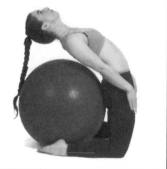

cat stretch

This is an effective stretch for all the muscles of your back. It's not only beneficial at the end of a core workout, it's also quite soothing after a long period of sitting.

STARTING POSITION: Kneel behind the ball. Place your hands on top of the ball, rolling it forward until your arms are straight. Your pelvis should be tucked slightly so that your body forms a straight line from your shoulders to your knees. Press the tops of your feet against the floor. **INHALE** and push down on the ball.

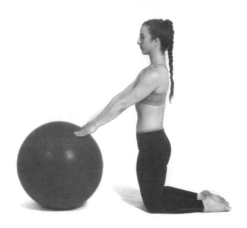

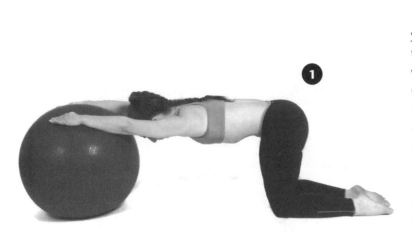

1 As you **EXHALE**, bend forward from your hips, extending your head, neck and spine into a tabletop (flat) position. (The ball will roll forward as you bend.) Continuing to press down on the ball with your hands, slowly roll it out farther until you feel a stretch in your shoulders and back. Your hips and knees remain aligned; don't sit back on your ankles. To really get a good spinal stretch, think about lifting your head off of your neck and lengthening your tailbone down through your pelvis. Hold the outstretched position, relaxing your shoulders and feeling their weight opening and widening your back.

overhead torso stretch

Arching your back, like you do in this stretch, compresses and opens your spinal discs. The ball is a great tool for stretching your back since it provides support, making stretching safer.

STARTING POSITION: Sit on the ball with your hands at your sides, palms pressing down on the ball for support. Slowly walk your feet forward until your back is draped over the ball. The ball should support the natural curvature of your lower back. Your legs are hip-width apart, knees bent and feet flat on the floor. Let your head drop back and rest your hands on the front of your hips.

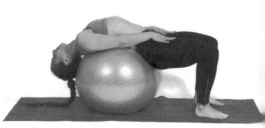

1

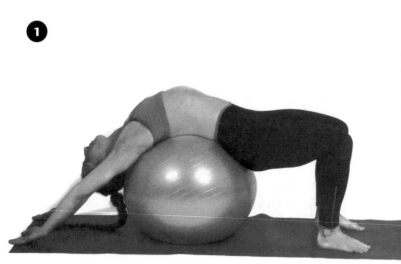

1 Extend your arms by your ears and reach back until you feel a stretch in your abs and back. Think about extending your fingers to touch the wall behind you. Concentrate on the curve of your spine sinking into the curve of the ball. Allow the weight of your neck and body to melt into the ball. Hold the stretch for 15 to 30 seconds.

TO COME OUT: Bend your legs and bring your arms to the sides of the ball. Slowly lower yourself into a seated position on the floor.

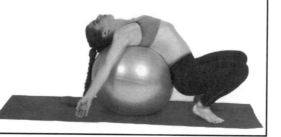

kneeling side stretch

This stretch will elongate your spine extensors and obliques, as well as every other muscle in your back and abs. You should feel the stretch through the entire side of your body.

STARTING POSITION: Kneel with your right hip next to the ball. Place your right hand on the far side of the ball. Extend your left leg straight out to your side and place the foot flat on the floor. Your left knee should face forward.

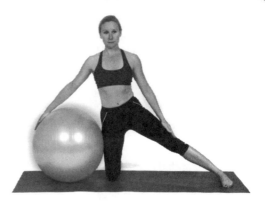

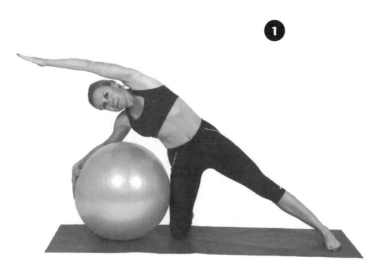

1 Extend your left arm straight over your head and reach toward the right side of the room. Keep both hips stacked atop each other, facing forward, and don't allow your pelvis to shift forward or back as you hold the stretch.

TO COME OUT: Push off the floor with your bent knee and bottom hand to return to the starting position.

seated side stretch

Everyday activities like carrying groceries or working at a computer can cause one side of your back to become tighter than the other. Performing side stretches can help you maintain balance by releasing tension.

STARTING POSITION: Sit on the ball with your legs hip-width apart and feet flat on the floor. Relax your arms along your sides. Contract your abs and press your pelvis slightly forward to put your spine in a neutral position. Your head, shoulders and butt are aligned.

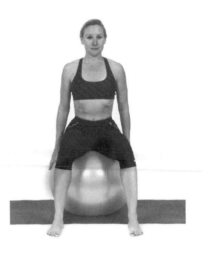

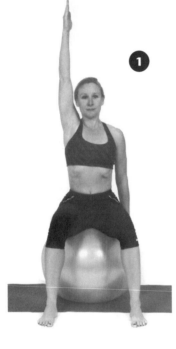

1 INHALE and raise your right arm straight overhead, palm facing in. As you **EXHALE**, lift through the side of the raised arm.

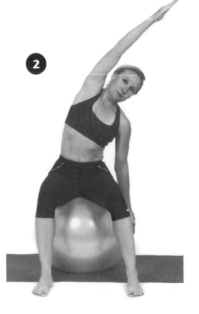

2 Keeping your lower body completely still, pull your arm over to the side so that your upper body leans toward your left. Keep your head and neck aligned with your shoulders even as you lean, and your back should not be arched. Relax your neck and allow your head to follow the sideways motion. Your left hand travels down the side of the ball and your right arm extends overhead. Hold the stretch.

This modified version of a yoga pose will strengthen your spine as it increases flexibility.

STARTING POSITION: Drape your body over the ball. Extend your legs straight out behind you and open them about hip width. Pull your toes back so that the balls of your feet are on the floor. Place your palms in front of you on the ball and rest your forearms against it, keeping your shoulders aligned with your elbows.

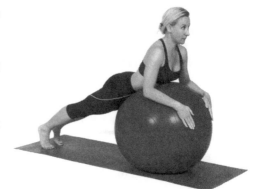

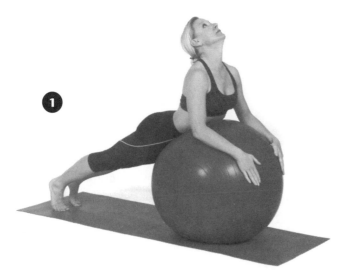

1 Keeping your head and neck in a neutral position, **INHALE** as you slowly curl your torso back, drawing your shoulder blades down your back to open your chest and lifting your head to elongate your neck. Don't arch too far back—stop at the point where you feel mild tension. Pause for one full breath.

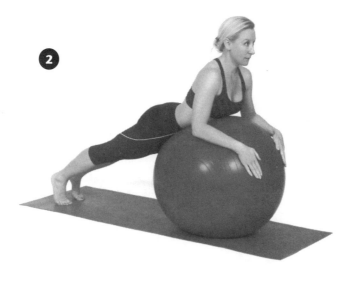

2 On an **EXHALE**, slowly lower your torso to the ball. Pause for a full breath before repeating.

spinal twist

This rotating stretch relieves tension in your lower back. The straighter your legs are, the deeper the stretch. As you advance, decrease the bend in your knees until you are performing the stretch with straight legs.

STARTING POSITION: Lie on your back with your legs bent, the ball between them, and your feet flat on the floor. Squeeze the ball with your thighs and knees to hold it in place. Extend your arms out to the sides into a T and press your palms flat into the floor. **INHALE** and contract your abs to help stabilize your body.

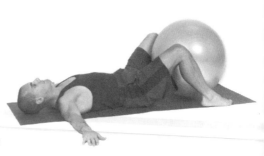

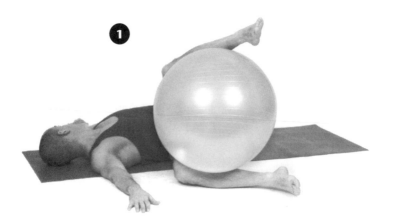

1 As you **EXHALE**, lift your legs and bring them to the right side of your body so that your right leg touches the floor and your left leg is above it, on top of the ball. Keep both shoulders pressed against the floor and turn your head toward your left side. If your shoulder is lifting, don't lower your bottom leg all the way to the floor. Hold the stretch for several breaths.

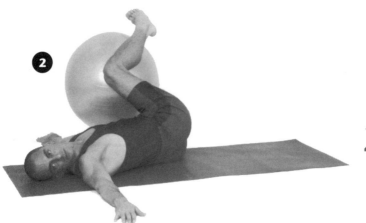

2 Return to center with control and repeat to the left side.

triangle stretch

This stretch is inspired by the downward-facing dog yoga pose. Besides your core, it stretches your shoulders, hamstrings and arms—many of the body parts you use during the workouts in this book.

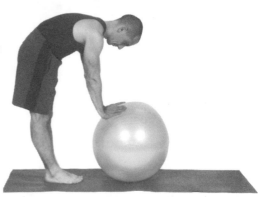

STARTING POSITION: Stand behind the ball with your legs together. Lean forward and place your palms on the part of the ball that's closest to you. **INHALE** and contract your abs.

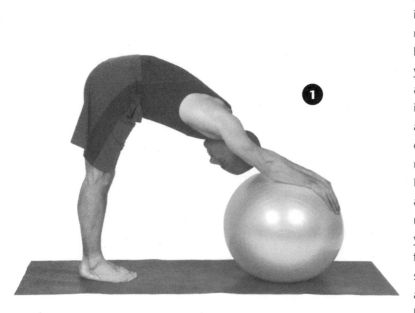

1 As you exhale, push the ball forward so that your arms are straight and extending out from your shoulders. Your back is elongated and your head is relaxed, but not hanging, between your arms (imagine your neck as the stick of a lollipop and keep your head stuck above it). Push your hips farther into the air and pull your shoulder blades down your back so that they're not hunched around your ears. Hold the stretch, glancing down at your belly once in a while to make sure it's not popping out. If your heels aren't pressed into the floor, that's okay. You can also slightly bend your legs, which will alleviate any discomfort in your hamstrings.

index

about the author

JEANINE DETZ earned bachelors degrees in English and psychology from Rutgers University. She's edited many health and fitness books for Weider Publications, including *Shape Do It Right*, *A Woman's Guide to Weight Training* and *Shape Lowfat & Easy Cookbook*. She has written for *Muscle & Fitness*, *Muscle & Fitness HERS*, *Weight Loss That Works*, *Flex* and *Shape*, and is currently articles editor at *Muscle & Fitness*. She also enjoys creative writing. Originally from Fair Lawn, New Jersey, Detz now resides in Los Angeles.

other books by ulysses press

ELLIE HERMAN'S PILATES MATWORK PROPS WORKBOOK: STEP-BY-STEP GUIDE WITH OVER 200 PHOTOS
Ellie Herman, $12.95
Explains how props can enhance Pilates: the magic circles tone arms, the small ball held between the legs shapes thighs, the foam roller stretches the chest and shoulders, and the large exercise ball builds core stability.

ELLIE HERMAN'S PILATES WORKBOOK ON THE BALL: ILLUSTRATED STEP-BY-STEP GUIDE
Ellie Herman, $13.95
Combines the powerful slimming and shaping effects of Pilates with the low-impact, high-intensity workout of the ball.

FIT IN 15: 15-MINUTE MORNING WORKOUTS THAT BALANCE CARDIO, STRENGTH, AND FLEXIBILITY
Steven Stiefel, $12.95
Fit in 15 details a unique, full-body fitness program that even the busiest person can work into a morning schedule. The fun and flexible "7 days/7 workouts" plan lets readers choose from 55 specially designed 15-minute workouts.

WEIGHTS ON THE BALL WORKBOOK: STEP-BY-STEP GUIDE WITH OVER 350 PHOTOS
Steven Stiefel, $14.95
With exercises suited for all skill levels, *Weights on the Ball Workbook* shows how to simultaneously use weights *and* a balance ball for the ultimate total-body workout.

To order these books call 800-377-2542 or 510-601-8301, fax 510-601-8307, e-mail ulysses@ulyssespress.com, or write to Ulysses Press, P.O. Box 3440, Berkeley, CA 94703. All retail orders are shipped free of charge. California residents must include sales tax. Allow two to three weeks for delivery.